Thirty-One Days to Healthy Sexual Relationships

A Contemplative's Field Manual to Guide Sexual Relationships

MARGARET PINDER,
LINDA CARLSON,
KAREN ISBELL

BALBOA.PRESS

A DIVISION OF HAY HOUSE

Balboa Press books may be ordered through booksellers or by contacting:

Balboa Press
A Division of Hay House
1663 Liberty Drive
Bloomington, IN 47403
www.balboapress.com
1 (877) 407-4847

Print information available on the last page.

ISBN: 978-1-9822-3805-6 (sc)
ISBN: 978-1-9822-3807-0 (hc)
ISBN: 978-1-9822-3806-3 (e)

Library of Congress Control Number: 2019917812

Balboa Press rev. date: 11/05/2019

Contents

From a Colleague who graciously agreed to review our book before its publication….

Margaret Pinder and Linda Carlson are the perfect people to write *Thirty-One Days to Radically Fulfilling Sexuality* because of their decades of counseling, teaching, and helping others to gain sexual maturity.

Both authors, through their teaching, counseling, and research, have impacted thousands of lives in the area of sexuality. Their passion for understanding sexual identity and expression, as well as their distinctive insights into busting myths about sexuality and revealing truths ring true in the pages of this book.

Margaret and Linda are two of the most important influences in my life and have taught me much about what it means to be a caring person who lives with no regrets. As colleagues and friends, they have shared their time and knowledge with me and have changed my life in many positive ways. I have witnessed their teaching on sexuality to groups and observed their compassion and commitment to helping others understand what it means to be fully alive as sexual beings and how to make positive life choices.

In Thirty-One Days, they provide a daily compass for your journey to sexual maturity. Their goal to comfort, challenge, and enlighten will inspire, and support the daily sexual decisions you face. Within each lesson, Margaret and Linda shatter many common assumptions about sexuality with a deeply human approach that is intuitive, practical, and real. The thirty minutes you spend each day learning, reflecting, and ultimately practicing what you gain from these pages is profound and life-changing.

Thirty-One Days to Healthy Sexual Relationships is one of the most important and captivating books I have ever read, full of meaning and powerful ideas. It will not only change the way you think of your sexuality; it might just change the way you live your life. May you embrace the fullness of your sexuality and experience more joy and fulfillment in each day of your future!

Authors Note: Dr. Jonathan Schultz, academic leader, professor, author, consultant, and mentor lives in Dallas, TX. As a fellow colleague, we know Jonathan to take seriously his study of healthy sexual relationships. We hold him in our deepest regard and know him to be filled with genuine, practical integrity.

Introduction

It seems a given: we cannot avoid our sexuality as adults. Much less certain is the extent to which we are prepared for this often terrifying arena! This field manual is our effort to guide you through the terrain in ways that will increase your likelihood for survival and success.

To begin, we encourage you to value your own perspective as a legitimate starting point. Each of our thirty-one thoughts or guidelines for your consideration can be relevant whether you have never been actively sexual or you have had multiple fitful starts and stops that have left you crying, "Uncle! No more!"

The following simple structure may be helpful: Please allow a minimum of thirty minutes in one sitting to read and reflect upon each day's lesson. During this time, allow yourself the luxury of being attentive, open, and receptive to any questions that may form.

You may choose to journal, to share with a confidante, or to be quietly introspective. Allow the affirmations to fill your mind, heart, body, and spirit with a vision of your sexual self today, whole and committed to positive living and loving.

Note: You may complete this manual on your own or within the setting of a small and carefully chosen group. As with sexual expression itself, there is more than one way to accomplish the goal!

Let's say that as you read the entry for Day One, you find that the information paints a rather grim view of how sexuality has been used and misused. Please don't be put off reading or stop reading.

We feel it is important to lay out the current state of affairs. Day One is offered so that the reader may understand what is at stake as we begin to raise our awareness and shift our intention. Sexuality is a given, and sexual power cannot be denied or minimized. We are either wise and care-filled in its expression or hurtful to ourselves and others. With this in mind, you will find that the remainder of the days focus on what you can do differently to create a *no-regrets future through intentional sexual decision-making.*

Please accept this field manual as an example of our own personal and professional learning as we, too, have been warriors in the arena of sexual relationships. We continue to draw from learning in this arena in ways that enrich our whole lives. We wish you the same kind of transformational learning!

With our deep regards,

Linda and Margaret, 2019, along with Karen Isbell, our deeply appreciated reader and contributor. Karen read every page, offered important edits, and wrote three contemplative questions and an affirmation for each chapter.

You Might Run from Your Sexuality, but You Can't Hide: From the Get-Go, Sexual Power Is a Part of Who You Are

Human history is also sexual history. So let's first take a look at what sexuality and human relations researchers and historians are telling us. We will see that we don't become sexual—we are sexual. History tells us that humans have sought sexual companionship and sexual expression in every society since the beginning of recorded history. Major ancient cultures, notably Middle Eastern, Hebraic, and Chinese cultures, are full of literature, sacred texts, and art extolling the virtues of sexuality and sexual relationships. And more recently, Pfizer conducted a global study of twenty-six thousand people in twenty-eight countries to find out how important sex was in their overall lives. The results were telling: 83 percent of men and 63 percent of women said that sex was very, extremely, or moderately important in their lives. Not surprisingly, in both women and men there was a strong relationship between their reported sexual well-being and their overall happiness.

As we can see from the above, this embedded desire we have for sexual expression and relational companionship seems to have both a cultural and a biological basis. For years, medical researchers and sex researchers have associated the release of oxytocin, a hormone produced in the brain, with the release of breast milk and mother–child bonding during breastfeeding. It is now thought that oxytocin has a similar effect on attraction and emotional bonding in couples. It plays a significant role during attraction, falling in love, sexual desire, sexual pleasure, and orgasm. Researchers have also discovered that people who seem to have a low ability to form affectionate and emotionally bonded relationships also have much lower levels of oxytocin. How appropriate then that oxytocin is also referred to as the love hormone!

Each of us has been imbued with a powerful life energy that reaches up and out, longing for acknowledgment and expression. This is eros. When repressed, this energy will come popping up somewhere else. Imagine a long, fully inflated balloon. If we press down on one end of the balloon, the air at that end gets moved or displaced to the other end of the balloon. Eros is like that. It cannot be destroyed, but it can be displaced or misplaced and thereby show up in a distorted fashion!

As best we can tell from history and the research into sexual expression and behavior, all ancient and contemporary societies had/have rules designed to regulate sexual behavior. Some of those rules, however, serve(d) to repress or restrict sexual conduct and sexual behavior, somewhat like the depressed-balloon example. For instance, many societies taught and still teach which sexual behaviors are appropriate for men and which are appropriate for women. In Western as well as Islamic and Chinese cultures, there has always been a theme of sex mainly serving the purpose of procreation. And some views of Christianity teach that sexuality is innately sinful unless practiced inside marriage. Even Saint Augustine, a fifth-century bishop, referred to sexuality as "the monster in the groin."

Some of the statistics around sexual distortions tell a very sad and challenging story. Take a look at these numbers:

- For FY 2018, a total of 7,500 sexual harassment claims were filed with the Equal Employment Opportunity Commission (EEOC). For 2015, a total of 6,822 charges of sexual harassment were reported by the EEOC. Of these, 17.1 percent were filed by males and 82.9 percent were filed by females.
- A US Department of Defense (DOD) study, anonymously conducted and compiled by the DOD every two years, showed that in FY 2018, about 20,500 service members across all branches were sexually assaulted. Of these 20,500 members, about 13,000 were women and about 7,500 were men.
- The DOD's "Annual Report on Sexual Assault in the Military" from May 1, 2018, reported the following:
    - Sexual assault increased by about 10 percent in FY 2017 across all four military branches.
    - FY 2017 had 6,769 reports of sexual assault.
    - FY 2018 had 7,623 reports of sexual assault.
- In an Office of Civil Rights investigation of 152 colleges for their handling of sexual violence claims, an increase of more than 400 percent was found.
- An Association of Universities report published in 2015—data from 2013—showed the following:
    - That 11.2 percent of all students experienced rape or sexual assault.
    - Among graduate and professional students, 8.8 percent of females and 2.2 percent of males experienced rape or sexual assault.
    - Among undergraduate students, 23.1 percent of females and 5.4 percent of males experienced sexual assault or rape.
- The organization End Rape on Campus (EROC) reported in 2019 that more than 50 percent of rapes on campus occurred during the first six to eight weeks of being on campus.

- Centers for Disease Control and Prevention data states that in 2014, 249,078 babies were born to girls and women aged fifteen to nineteen.
- Centers for Disease Control and Prevention data states that sexually transmitted diseases in people ages fifteen to twenty-four account for half of all new sexually transmitted infections. This age group makes up just over one-fourth of the sexually active population but accounts for half of the twenty million new infections.
- An April 2012 PEW Research Center survey of 1,197 self-identified lesbian, gay, bisexual, and transgender people found that 92 percent say society has become more accepting of them in the past decade. At the same time, about 39 percent of them say that at some point in their lives they were rejected by a family member or close friend because of their sexual orientation or gender identity.

How is it that on planet Earth we have developed this history of sexual violence? Are we helpless, or can we do something about it? Do we have any hope of turning things around?

We do have hope. Although sexuality may be wild and crazy, even destructive at times, it can also be a source of profound delight, joy, and nurturance.

Think of it this way: if there were no sexuality, none of us would be here. Sexuality is the bridge between our spirits or souls—our nonphysical essence—and our physical forms. At some point, two people decide to mate, and nine months or so later, as a result of this sexual union, a new creature emerges. And we keep doing this over and over, to the tune of about seven billion people on this tiny little planet. We are wired as sexual beings. And, thankfully, we are also wired to learn and to keep on learning.

Perhaps even more important than its role in our birth is sexuality's role in connecting us to each other. Otherwise, why would some people abandon family or fortune for the one they love? It is pleasure we seek when we risk it all to find and to hold on to that which we consider dear. Sexuality, in its many forms, draws us out of isolation. It is in our childhood play, in our fantasies, in our dreams of adult partnering, and in our major life decisions and course changes. So just what is this sexuality, this deep energetic pull?

We define sexuality this way: Sexuality, not to be located in just one part of our humanness, courses through body, mind, and soul to bring both deep pleasure and invigorating life to our whole being. Rather than set up residence solely in our genitals, sexuality, much like the wind, is the life energy that blows where it will, making or breaking lives depending upon its relationship with two other precious life capacities, wisdom and love. Sexuality evokes a mysterious alchemy in our lives; it can be both life-affirming and murderous depending upon the direction of our will and the presence of wisdom and maturity in our hearts and minds. It will not be boxed. It cannot be destroyed. This is its largeness. This is why we write about sexuality, and this is why we must become its students. Never will we possess sexuality, but if we do not embrace it, it will possess us—and that has serious consequences.

Questions for Reflection

1. How has the power of sexuality manifested itself in my life? How has it manifested in the lives of those I care about?
2. When have I seen it create bonds of love and experiences of safe, sensual pleasure, and when have I seen it destroy the dignity, esteem, and well-being of myself or others?
3. What factors seem to determine whether sexuality is manifested in a positive or a negative way?

Margaret Pinder, Linda Carlson, Karen Isbell

Affirmation

Sexuality is a powerful force working through my life. Only by developing maturity and harnessing my internal wisdom can I wield its power for good.

Become the Best Sexual Partner You Can Be

From birth, we are sexual creatures—albeit immature sexual creatures. Healthy sexuality at birth differs from adult sexuality. The difference is developmental. We are designed to grow, change, become, and mature. It is written in our human code. From infancy, we seek pleasure and want to avoid pain. Even from the first trimester of life, an infant seeks to self-soothe and to get the attention he or she needs for nurturance, sustenance, and comfort.

Within his or her family, a little one learns how to read the signs and the expectations. By the time the toddler walks and talks, patterns and impressions are formed. These imprints continue to be carried into adulthood. But besides the family, we are also impacted by other influences outside us: our schools, our neighborhoods, religious organizations, popular media, and high-impact social or environmental events such as a war or even a destructive hurricane or tornado. These external events often destabilize our communities and our daily lives.

Simultaneously, we experience internal pressures to mature and grow. Our brains continue developing and forming. Our bodies develop, hormones change, and emotional patterns form. Values, beliefs, and personal boundaries take shape. Then, with some predictability, we experience changes in sexual knowledge, awareness, and energy.

Together, these external and internal factors influence how we think, feel, and act and how we interpret our world. Then, as we go out into the world, we are faced with multiple kinds of decisions. For some decisions, we may feel prepared. For others, not so much. There will be times when, no matter what we do, things will not work out as we would like. Perhaps in no other arena than our sexuality do we find the choices and decisions more daunting. And to complicate the matter, there is a good chance that along the way our sexual teachers have not been particularly well prepared or forthcoming. So we keep moving forward with our sexuality clumsily, at times falling down then getting up and muddling through.

Starting out, we don't have all the answers around our sexuality, but what if the following were true?

- Before we acted on our sexual wants and desires, we asked the question, "How will this affect the other person and me afterward?"
- When we made a mistake or hurt someone else sexually, we were able to forgive ourselves or the other person.
- We were able to wait to have sexual experiences until we either had birth control or we were ready to risk getting pregnant and raising a child.
- We were able to learn how to protect ourselves from contracting a sexually transmitted disease.
- We were able to find our way through the awkwardness of learning to be sexually active by dealing with the mixed emotions and the inevitable hurts.

If we can imagine moving through our lives with courage, openness, and willingness to learn, then we can create such a life and a world.

The following table identifies the stages of our sexual development. Just as our body, brain, and morality develops, so does our sexuality.

Use this chart as a guide when seeking to understand sexuality and making sexual decisions along the way:

Sexual stages of development	Possible experiences
Using all senses to experience pleasure (vs. pain)	Responding to either comfort (with laughing, excitement, smiling, cooing, movement, self-soothing) or discomfort (with struggle or crying).
Mutual exchanges and play	Normal, nonaggressive exploration of others' bodies and one's own body. Kinds of play and exploration depict unique personality styles. Atypical actions may also be learned.
Curious inquiry	Asking questions about the meaning of our sexual body parts, sensations, and boundaries in relationships. Healthy curiosity and sexuality develop provided caregivers provide physical, emotional, and relational safety.
Sexual practices, both inherited and adopted	Sexual actions and behaviors now reflect personal preferences and self-awareness. Role of family and culture becomes more evident as the child learns through imitation, adoption of cultural practices, and personal choices. A tension exists between a shame-based sexuality and respect-based sexuality. For many, this is the final stage of sexual development.
Cultivated desire	The "want" for sexual feelings and activities shows up. Our life energy seeks more pleasure, joy, delight, play, and appreciation. Sexuality becomes art and beauty. Our sexual practices honor all participants.

Sacred initiation into sexual mysteries	A shift occurs from not merely "wanting" to "giving." Conscious giving of self to the other in a mutual "holding" of each other: intimacy. A new level of intimacy emerges as we mutually and willingly give to one another sexually. Sexuality at this stage is rarely, if ever, destructive because we now experience self and other with extraordinary respect and value.
Continued discovery, awakening, and compassion	Now changed by previous sacred sexual experiences, we enter into new sexual experiences in ways characterized as both humble and bold, spontaneous and caring, life-giving and life-receiving. Most people who reach this level of sexual experience agree that it is not a continuous state of being. Rather we experience moments of bliss, awe, and oneness within the context of our daily lives.

Our hope is that as you read through the chart and think about your sexuality and life energy, you envision yourself as a sexually awakened person who honors both yourself and your partner. If we continue to learn about ourselves and our sexuality, the pleasures will abound.

On the other hand, if, as you consider this vision, you find it too daunting or complex, we encourage you to find a trusted adult with whom you can discuss your questions. Should you not know anyone with whom you can talk, please read on. Also, listen to and trust yourself, your intuition, and your insights. If you are currently facing an obvious or highly likely sexual risk, take precautions. Avoid the situation if you can, or at least until you can develop a plan for safety. Most cities and counties have rape crisis centers that have 24/7 online access. Other online 24/7 options are available when one is in crisis. State and local counseling organizations have lists of prepared counselors. County family court services list appropriate local resources. In addition, many local community resources such as churches, local physicians or nurse practitioners, and family law practices are available for consultation. Or in the event of an immediate crisis, local emergency services, either transport or local emergency rooms, may be of assistance.

From Day One and Day Two you should have surmised that we consider sexuality to be among our most precious gifts and traits, not to be hidden, misused, or experienced as shame. With courage and wise decision-making, you can create life-giving sexual memories that will bring joy to you as you later reflect upon your life. You will also have the pleasure of knowing that you brought much joy to your sexual partner(s).[1] Take good care of your sexuality.

Questions for Reflection

1. To what degree have I experienced and/or expressed respect and honor for my sexual partner(s) in my life?
2. To what degree have I acted with a mature sense of caution and care for the safety and integrity of my own physical body and the body of my partner?

---

[1] By using the plural when talking about partners, we are not suggesting simultaneous multiple partners. Rather, we acknowledge that given greater longevity for many more people, adults will become divorced or widowed and will most likely have more than one sexual partner in their lifetime.

Also, while we do not recommend having affairs or sexual experiences for recreation or without intimacy, we acknowledge that these types of experiences do occur. They can be powerful teachers if we actively choose to learn from them and own our part in them.

3. To what degree have I allowed myself to experience and enjoy my sexuality as a force that is larger than the desire and pleasure experienced by my sexual anatomy?

Affirmation

I become a better sexual partner when I remember to begin any sexual expression from a space of respect for myself and my partner.

Realize that You can Learn Something from Every Sexual Experience You Have

These days we hear a lot about experiential learning. People whose lives shout happiness, empowerment, and abundance tend to be people who live life large. They aren't armchair quarterbacks. Not just talking about things, they have some skin in the game.

With sexuality, it is the same. If our goal is to live out a sexuality that brings joy, confidence, and titillating fantasies and experiences that linger long after they have occurred in real time, then we must pay the price of saying yes when saying no might be easier. We must become committed to something beyond where we've been. We must get up, get intimate, get serious, get conscious, and get involved in helping others learn how to be passionately and compassionately sexual as well.

The price we pay is letting go of fear and control. Rich, abundant sexuality requires courage, hope, grit, and a willingness to fail but also a commitment to keep on trying. And ultimately a rich and rewarding sexuality requires that we trust the process, seeing ourselves as purposeful beings who are here to live fully and generously. We think about such things as the following:

- Who am I?
- With whom do I talk about sexuality?

- With whom do I experience my sexuality?
- Will my sexual experience be consistent with someone else's?
- What kinds of sexual experiences do I enjoy or even love?
- Can I continue to belong to my group if/when/as I experience my sexuality?
- What happens if I disappoint people who are important to me in terms of how I experience my sexuality?
- Are there ways my sexuality and my life's work intersect and/or affect one another?
- When I die, what kind of sexual legacy will I leave behind?

Throughout all of history, in every land and every tradition, people have sorted themselves into two groups: those who find a way through tough circumstances and those who fail to see their way through. And in the end, no matter the specific details, the one thing that seems most predictive of who will thrive is the person's willingness to show up, to get involved, and to just do something that shifts the energy and the system toward greater resilience and capacity.

This "showing up" could be called "going with the flow," "being aligned," "living in the now," or "being present," but whatever we call it, the showing up will always expose us, either to ourselves or to others. And once we are seen, we can never again fully deny our existence.

This one aspect of our sexuality alone makes it one of our most important teachers. We can run and we can hide, but ultimately we cannot escape the fact that we exist.

To the contrary, if we see and hear our sexuality as it shows up / manifests, we increase the likelihood that we will also face ourselves in all the other important aspects of being human.

Sexuality, while fraught with obstacles, disappointments, and pain, as well as pleasure, can take us where we want to go in terms of the very human traits of humility, courage, genuineness, empowerment, wisdom, and even love.

Does this mean that we need to naively set out to have as many sexual experiences as possible? No, it does not. But it does mean that we need to hold our sexuality in high esteem. Thus, much like a servant who enters the chamber of a lord, we spend more time preparing to enter the chamber than we will spend in the chamber. To bring honor to ourselves, we must respect that our sexuality is among our most sacred and most powerful gifts and seek to bring it honor as we consciously, reflectively act sexually for the purpose of beauty, goodness, and truth.

Depending upon our circumstances, relationships, and developmental level, any of the following sexual acts may be legitimate. Under different circumstances, any of the same acts could be considered illegitimate:

- masturbation in one's own bedroom
- celibacy while focused on a sports contest
- fantasies of wild exotic sexual practices with one's sexual partner
- sexual intercourse four or five times a day
- sexual pleasuring of each other without any genital penetration.

In summary, Day Three invites us to value our sexual experiences as life teachers. Consider that if we adopt one pattern or approach to our sexual behavior, never changing or reflecting upon it to learn from it, our sexuality becomes stagnant, compulsive. The alternative is messy and often takes us into awkward, even painful, experiences, but it is the path of learning and transformation.

Questions for Reflection

1. What are one or two lessons I have learned from my sexual experiences so far in my life?
2. How have I played a role in teaching important life lessons to others through my/our expressions of my/our sexuality?
3. How can the lessons I have learned through my sexuality bring benefits to other aspects of my life and the lives of others?

Affirmation

Sexuality is a sacred gift, not only because of the pleasure it gives me but also because of the lessons it can teach me throughout my life.

Acknowledge and Accept Responsibility for Your Patterns of Sexual Behavior

Gradually patterns of sexual practice form. These range from addictive or avoidant patterns to fully conscious, healthy, compassionate patterns.

From the time we are born, we have a relationship with pleasure and pain. As little sensory infants, we learn quickly to smile and goo because people respond well to these signals. And when we cry and scream, people around us become agitated and do all sorts of things designed to make us stop crying. So our relationship with power and influence is born. And later, usually even before preschool, we discover that not all body parts are the same. When we touch certain parts of our body, it feels good. Other parts of the body are not so responsive, so those patterns of touch aren't reinforced. In addition, we take in and are influenced by messages from our caregivers. But that's not all. Already as individuals we show unique types of responses to our outer world, and we initiate in various ways as well.

Among the energies that we have is sexual energy, also known as our libidinal energy. This energy never leaves us, even though we will learn lots of different ways to express it. Some of us will make friends with our sexuality, but far more often we find that our sexual experiences exceed our understanding of what they mean, our ability to know how to deal with them, or how they affect both us and the others involved.

Herein lies the problem. Fearing that our sexuality exceeds our capacity to control it, we create layers of defenses to avoid thinking about it. "Owning it"—well, what is that? A whole range of defenses is possible. For example, one person might adhere to a strict code of repression, avoiding all sexual contact or conversations about sexuality, whereas another person might flaunt her sexuality, which could be her defensive way of making this her primary sexual identity. In either case, fear and anxiety are the driving behavior. Instead of having a "sex positive" identity, the two examples show a "shame and defend" sexual identity. And to add to your understanding of the genesis of these identities, know that identities typically are formed by the time we are in our teens. Neither of these identities, however, allows for healthy discussions that lead to meaningful exploration, mutual consideration, and guilt-free choices that can be both playful and full of integrity.

So how can we develop the type of relationship with our sexuality that generates a healthy sexual identity?

Let's first describe what a sexually addictive personality looks like, and then we'll describe what a sexually empowered, compassionate identity looks like.

Having a sexually addictive personality means that we rate our sexuality and ourselves based upon the frequency of our sexual experiences, the magnitude of physical pleasure experienced, and the perception of attractiveness that is derived from exuding this type of persona/image. The more intense and more exotic, the better; this has been the gold standard in our culture. So it leads to always seeking more, more, more. These acquisitions (i.e., sexual encounters) become the substance of choice.

In contrast, a sex-positive identity is derived from a balance between *purpose*, *discipline*, and *integrity* in relationships.

First, let's look at purpose. When we have a clear purpose in life, keeping certain values in perspective and acting intentionally toward our goals and with goodwill toward others, we will approach our sexuality in terms of how it affects our whole life. Second, we work to consistently make decisions that foster success, joy, and peace instead of ones that create some form of dysfunction or disorder. This is discipline. Equally important is the third characteristic of a sex-positive identity, integrity. This kind of self-awareness embodies thoughts, feelings, actions, and relationships that reflect a personal commitment that goes way beyond an attitude of just "What's in it for me?"

A sexual identity that embodies a high level of self-awareness, ownership, intention, care, appreciation, and compassion tends to produce sexual experiences of equal merit and creates relationships that last well beyond one or two experiences.

Regardless of where one finds oneself on a path, it is possible to change paths and become more sex positive. But it should be noted that changing course sooner rather than later can prevent much pain and regret. In addition, it can be helpful to remember that learning is social. Yes, as individuals we must change from within, but rarely, if ever, do we make lasting, transformative changes without meaningful engagement with at least one other person. Is this risky? Yes. Is it worth it? Yes. Is it easy? No.

Find your courage. Make your commitment. Find at least one trusted teacher/coach/mentor/friend. Keep learning. Finish the next sentence with a sex-positive message: "I am ______________!"

Take inventory of your motivation, goals, and intentions—how you decide to approach sexuality. Conduct a review of the following:

- Frequency
- Intensity
- Style
- Play/compulsions
- Choice of partner(s)
- Gender choices
- Patterns of thinking
- Identity ownership
- Power in sexuality
- Before, during, and after—what does it look like?
- Hide or talk about?
- Shame
- Multiple partners
- Toys
- Supportive family
- Consistency both internally and externally
- Reputation
- Character
- Awareness
- Fantasies
- Turning points
- Feedback
- Bartering with sexuality
- Lead with sex and/or hide sexuality?
- Best practices

Questions for Reflection

1. What forces do you feel influenced your sexual identity?
2. Do you feel that you have ever tended toward an extreme of sexual shame and repression or sexual flamboyance and rebellious acting out? If so, how did these behaviors and attitudes affect your sexual identity?

Affirmation

I am responsible for how I express my sexuality. Instead of coming from a place of shame or selfishness, my sexuality can reflect the integrity of who I am.

Day Five

Examine Ways Your Sexual Decision-Making Affects Your Life and Relationships

If we come to know and own our sexuality, we will increase our chances of reducing sexual stress, including anxiety and poor decision-making.

The following table, "Seven levels of sexual decision-making—doing what is good," describes sexual behaviors and their associated desires. For each level we have described a sexual behavior and the desire associated with that behavior. In other words, each behavior is trying to get a need met. The more we understand the motivation behind the behavior, the more conscious our decisions become. The table is arranged from the lowest level of ethical sexual decision-making to the highest level of ethical sexual decision-making. As we have said before, throughout our lives we develop across multiple dimensions. Consider, then, that our sexual decision-making can also develop.

Seven levels of sexual decision-making—doing what is good

Vicious use of sexual force to release strong energy/emotions without regard for pain inflicted on the other	Avoid separateness	Rape, violent sexual assault
Lazy/convenient use of an available other to satisfy release of sexual tension	Comfort and diversion	One-night stand
Psychologically rationalized participation in sexual behavior, either initiating or receiving	Anesthetize and minimize the internal conflict	Sexual behavior when one knows it is not good decision-making
Recreational sexual behavior with intentional effort to respect self and other; little or no regard for any deeper/integral meaning of sexuality	Affirmation and validation from external source	Friends with benefits
Regard for sexuality as a connected meaningful part of one's whole self; careful choices about sexual practices	Consistency between internal and external; to know and to be known intimately	Making conscious, intentional choices as to when and with whom one has sex, most often within the context of a committed relationship

Deep regard for sexuality as a powerful expression of one's eros: conscious, practiced engagement in sexual behavior	To use one's will to be honorable and excellent in one's sexual behavior	Two coworkers find each other extremely attractive but choose to refrain from sexual engagement because they realize, and discuss the fact, that it is not in either's best interests
Recognition that sexuality is entrusted/given from a source beyond the self but given directly to the individual self, who has a moral responsibility in terms of if, when, and how the gift is released, shared, or experienced	To surrender one's will to be a part of, even one with, the creative source and the sexual partner at the same time	Two committed sex partners come together to actively give each other the form of sexual pleasure most pleasing to each other

Do you believe that we can mature in our sexual decision-making? If we own our sexuality, will we make better decisions? Will we experience lower or higher levels of sexual anxiety?

While a simple answer might be nice, the reality is that it is not a one-step process. We do not jump from no sexual experience or a low degree of learning about our sexuality to arrive at a place of sexual maturity. However, if we stay the course through our youth and adulthood, we can mature our sexuality. To arrive at a place where our internal sexual perceptions and definitions are consistent with our external sexual experiences and relationships, we must do the following:

- consciously raise our awareness of how sexuality works,
- identify how intimacy is developed and sustained, and

- observe how we transfer our learning about sexuality to other dimensions of being human.

We arrive at a place of sexual well-being not because we do everything right or follow a certain code but because we are willing to look at ourselves along the way. We ask the tough questions in terms of examining our roles in our relationships. This means we recognize that in any situation, the truth is arrived at by looking at multiple perspectives instead of choosing sides and holding tenaciously to the one that supports only our biases. We must move about the relationship considering all perspectives with respect and reasonable attention.

Only when we listen to our own voice, as well as to others' voices, are we ready to declare what we know. This is not always easy, for we may hold wildly and widely different views of what has happened or is happening. Also, we may be aware of consequences or sociopolitical reasons for which one perspective is more attractive than another. Then, if we consider any power differentials, our levels of fear may rise and self-protection may supersede telling the truth. So, you see, owning one's sexuality is often a complicated matter. And because this is so, our anxiety may skyrocket as we attempt to gain sexual integrity and maturity. The following two examples show how anxiety and growth are intertwined:

Let's say that you want to have sex with your boyfriend, but your mother has forbidden you to use birth control measures. You start college in the fall and do *not* want to get pregnant. Also, you know two young women who have recently contracted herpes, and you are afraid to ask your boyfriend if he can show you that he is sexually "clean." Not only that, but also, even though you are technically a virgin, you have not discussed your sexual practices with your physician. Anxiety, fear? Probably.

Or you may find yourself excited about a new job, only to discover that your new boss has a history of and reputation for sexual harassment. You've been at the new job approximately three weeks before he approaches you at the end of the day, requesting that you join him for drinks on your way home. You and your partner have plans. What questions must you ask (and answer) to ensure your decision is consistent with a higher level of decision-making?

Questions for Reflection

1. How has anxiety about my sexuality and sexual expression affected my decisions in the past?
2. How does anxiety about my sexuality and sexual expression affect me today?
3. How does the anxiety I have felt or am feeling around my sexuality become transformed into wisdom and sound decision-making?

Affirmation

I can move from stress and anxiety to integrity in my sexuality only when I take the time to reflect before I act, ensuring my sexual actions express my true beliefs, priorities, and commitments.

Dare to Bring Your Full Goodness, both Emotional and Physical, to Your Partner in the Present Encounter

Sexual intimacy requires that a person contain her or his anxiety while expressing his or her authentic self. It is a *learned* capacity that requires vulnerability, curiosity, empathy, and humble audacity.

Think about one or two people whom you respect and want to spend time with. Chances are that these people or this person is someone who, when you're together, is totally present with you. He or she does not fidget, or reaching for his or her cell phone, or compete with you for the next word. This person seems calm, listens, and responds to what you say in ways that show you that he or she hears you deeply.

We all need people like this in our worlds. Too, we all need to become this kind of person for others, for it is this "living presence" that best describes love in action. If you or I can't spend time with someone, then we can't truly say that we are actively loving them. We may have well-meaning sentiments toward them, but this is not actualized love.

Throughout history, people have defined love. We even have multiple kinds of love defined:

- Agape—divine love
- Eros—sensual, holistic connectivity love
- Phileo—the nonsexual love of friendship

But one of the best definitions of love, it seems to us, comes from Erich Fromm, written over half a century ago. In *The Art of Loving*, Fromm defines love as an art, suggesting that we not only find meaning in love but also that we practice being loving. In other words, our expressions of love must move beyond words; love must show up in our actions—but not just any actions. Fromm lays out four characteristics that will always be present in love: (1) knowledge, (2) respect, (3) responsibility, and (4) care. We would add a fifth: truth.

Actually, love is our true state of being. It is the core of who we are because it is the part of God or the life force that shows up in our body, our personality, and our lifetime. (If coming from Judaism, Christianity, or Islam, you may express this connection in similar ways. Or if coming from a Buddhist or Hindu perspective, you may express things a bit differently.) Regardless of our major ways of knowing our source, we as humans are each spiritual beings having human experiences. We have an integral and indivisible connection to our depth.

If we are afraid to own our true core, then it is anxiety or fear that shows up. *Note:* We acknowledge that there are times when we discern in someone else an actual intent to harm us or others, and we must decide how to respond. In these times of high risk for violence, we must decide whether it is best to return violence for violence or if it is better/wiser to use nonviolent means to respond. This obviously includes times when the offender might choose a sexual behavior to inflict the harm. Much could be (and needs to be) said on this topic.

Our goal is to respond to life from a place of wholeness and presence. This doesn't mean that we will never be fearful or anxious. Our anxiety may be in proportion to our unpreparedness to act effectively. Each situation presents for the purpose of learning and not for the purpose of judgment.

Our goal is to grow into love, which is the antidote for anxiety. And if we set this as our goal, submitting to daily practices that teach us more and more about it, then we do find our way to full-bodied, robust presence.

Remember, Fromm discussed love as an art both in theory and in practice. The practice is required, and like the process of creating a fine wine, love requires time and patience, commitment to the process, and surrender to natural states of being that, paradoxically, require conscious cultivation. These necessary states of being include the following:

- Vulnerability
  Vulnerability cannot be circumvented. Without risk, there cannot be a full realization of our highest sexuality.
- Curiosity
  Curiosity is forever renewing itself in the human mind. It honors eros by seeking new life, including sexual life.
- Empathy
  Empathy invites sexual kindness and generosity where before there was aggression or indifference toward the sacred presence of the other.
- Humble audacity
  This is the fragrance of fully present, compassionate, passionate sexuality.

Questions for Reflection

1. To what degree have I experienced the fullness of my own presence while experiencing or exercising my sexuality with a partner?
2. To what degree have I acknowledged and honored the presence of my partner during our sexual experiences?
3. In what ways can I invite and cultivate a fuller experience of presence, my own and my partner's, as we relate to each other's sexuality?

Affirmation

My sexuality becomes an expression of true love as I both surrender and commit to the precious, sacred presence of my own embodied life force and the equally wondrous mystery of my partner.

Day Seven

Set Your Intention to Express Your Sexuality with Beauty and Gratitude

At its pinnacle, sexual practice is an exquisite form of artistry reflecting full, robust expressions of beauty and gratitude.

The statement above is firmly planted in paradox. For example:

- Beautiful sex cannot be hurried. Ah, but imagine this: In a busy supermarket, you suddenly feel someone's presence. You look up, your eyes catching the eyes of a stranger, and for a second, as your eyes meet, you zoom deep within the attractive stranger and feel an equal rush as the stranger penetrates any notion of boundaries that you may possess. Your entire day becomes charged with an energy that affirms and heightens your pleasure.
- You've been working all day. You're exhausted, but as you fall into bed, your partner begins stimulating your genital area. Groaning inside, you submit to the physical stimulation. It won't last long, and then sleep will come. Each of you brings the other to orgasm. No kisses are exchanged, no warm hugs. Just two orgasms and then sleep.

Both encounters are brief, and both are stimulating, but each is very different in the extent to which it arouses your whole being. And both types of sexual encounters hold value. But an entire life of either one or the other would be left wanting if that were the only type of sexual encounter one had.

Today's reading is about the kind of sexuality that arouses you, surrounds you, and sustains your whole being in pleasure and appreciation. Not only would it be arrogant to think that this type of sexuality could be served up as fast food, but also it would be futile.

Consider that your thirtieth wedding anniversary is six months away. One day as you ride the train to work, you see an advertisement for special holiday packages to multiple cities. Wasting no time, you begin your research to see if it is possible for the two of you to go away for at least three or four days.

As you pore over websites and make a few dozen phone calls, you locate what you think will be just the place. You are having a ball exploring ways to create a perfectly romantic and renewing week with the one you have come to love even more than you thought you could ever love anyone.

You create a separate bank account in which you make monthly deposits to grow the balance to a sizable amount before your anniversary trip. In addition, you coordinate closely with the manager of a locally owned and operated cottage to prearrange several surprises and special services. Among the ones you are most excited about are the personal, in-the-room massages and the fresh meals of local fruits, vegetables, seafood, and healthy beverages to be enjoyed in the late morning of your first full day in the country.

Wanting your anniversary sexual experiences to be tantalizing while also feeling completely natural, you arrange for a well-stocked kitchen, along with an array of fresh linens and at least three complete sets of bedroom attire for each of you to try on and purchase if you like. All these preparations reinforce that you have, as a couple, been transported away from anything mundane or demanding to a paradise for two where every need is met with complete beauty and grace and exquisite attention to detail.

Arriving on day one, you are met with the cottage manager, whom you have instructed to meet you with the package wrapped in plain brown paper, which he is to give you with verbal instructions to open and read aloud upon entering your private cottage. You graciously, attempting to portray innocence, accept the package and follow the manager to your abode.

Arriving, you notice a prominently displayed book along with chilled wine, chocolates, and finger sandwiches. Fresh robes lie open on the bed, and the windows have been opened so that you smell the fragrances of fresh flowers growing just below your windows.

Taking your lover by the hand, you lead her to the edge of the bed and, standing beside the bed, hold her close to you, walking toward the book.

You speak.

> "Notice that on this small side table there is a mysterious book. Perhaps it will guide us through our time here. Look, something is written on its cover: *Lover's Retreat: To Be Read One Day at a Time.*"

> Your lover agrees to this condition, and you proceed, reading only Day One: Awaken at will. Massages provided by local masseuse and masseur. All foods served in the room. Soak in tub or lie on the beach. Completely a no-demand day. No sexual intercourse, but plenty of touch.

Arising on Day Two, you read the following: "Visit to local florist to select an assortment of fresh flowers," which flowers will be arranged in a special vase that you have had pre-shipped to the florist for this occasion.

The florist experience is followed by a private breakfast in the courtyard of a small private bakery. Following breakfast, you return to your room, where you find your bed turned down, and on it are lying new lounge clothes for each of you plus an interesting-looking package marked, "Open only if ready to journey back through your partnership through the eyes of a perennially optimistic and devoted lover" (otherwise called a "gratitude journal," laced with visual and narrative memories). The remainder of the day follows your intentions. Still no genital intercourse.

On Day Three, the final day of your retreat vacation, you read the following:

"My love, this third day of our retreat brings me to my knees. Quite simply, I adore you and appreciate you. During the years we've had together, and during these past two days, you have graciously allowed me to pleasure you. Now, today, I come again with the full intention of loving you. Please grant me the pleasure of bringing you full ecstasy. To do so, I am yours. If you will, my dear, please allow me to approach and come with me to our marriage bed, our altar prepared for us to unite as one, with only one witness—the One within who makes us, calls us, and joins us and who will lead us forward in holy matrimony. Our oneness is our sacred prayer.

In this scenario, we see one man declare his love through his sexual/libinal/creative energy for his life partner. This type of sexuality is possible, but it requires that we commit and follow through in the following ways:

- We dare to declare that this is what we want.
- We discipline ourselves to stay focused on this type of sexual experience.
- We say no to setting our intention as anything less while acknowledging that practice is essential.
- We are clear about our sexual commitments to any potential sexual partner.
- We consistently and intently study the great literature and/or art on sexuality from multiple cultures, attempting to synthesize our learning across historical, cultural, philosophical, and scientific boundaries.
- We engage in honest, open dialogue about sexuality with others to learn about a sexuality that exists for the highest good of all involved.
- We develop self-awareness as a sexual being that is systemic, meaning that it includes close, honest surveys of our sexual history, our current sexual practices, and our vision for the future.
- We expand our self-awareness to include our developmental level; cultural relationships; daily calendar; family, community, and work-related circumstances; possibilities; worldview; and degree of empowerment.
- We develop specific sexually oriented rituals and regularly practice them to cultivate an appreciation for our creative legacy and potential.

- We learn gratitude practices around sexual themes through submission to regular times of meditation and overt manifestation.

When held carefully and consciously, the foregoing practices teach us that our sexuality has been planted within us to quicken our spirits and our bodies toward one another. We are wired for community. But in being difficult to build, community requires everything of us. To achieve and to sustain community requires that a power much greater than ourselves draw us out of our narcissism to care for more than ourselves and to honor the fact that life is meant for more than duty. We must have beauty to be fully human. Sexuality, while it can be ruthless and wild, is also filled with great beauty that, if appreciated, will help to carry us home.

Questions for Reflection

1. What experiences can you recall of being totally swept away by the beauty of something or someone in the world?
2. What words would you use to describe these experiences?
3. To what degree have your sexual experiences included an experience and appreciation of beauty, wonder, and gratitude?

Affirmation

The full expression of my sexuality begins with my ability to witness and enjoy the beauty of the world. The more open I am to the beauty that surrounds me every day, the more deeply I am able to see and appreciate the beauty that is in me and in my partner.

Recognize Patterns of Sexual Aggression in Yourself and Others

There is widespread agreement that this is a serious time with sexual violence reaching epidemic proportions. Thankfully victims of violence are speaking up. They are also linking arms to create effective countermeasures.

There is an awakening across multiple diverse groups of society with a growing body of evidence that shows people are actively learning both peacemaking and nonviolence as ways of life.

To conquer violence, we must see it from a close, upfront, and personal perspective. This doesn't mean that we must volunteer to be violated, but it does mean that we acknowledge that when one or more of us is violated, we all are. We are all victims until there are no victims, including the ones we call perpetrators, for they too have gone astray from their highest good, beauty, and empowerment.

When we are both brave and empathic, then we can hold our fellow humans' pain. We can see through their defenses to the fear and pain. Furthermore, we can resolve to help others become less isolated and alone. Therefore, we must learn to recognize violence in ourselves and in others—not so that we can guilt one another or join in pity parties, but so we can reveal, one person at a time, over and over again, our own and others' brilliance, hopes, dreams, and potential.

Sexual violence in all forms, as in the following examples, can be effectively dealt with. But first it must be seen and named. It must be operationally defined / walked out in terms of what it looks like. Each item in this list is an example of sexual violence:

- withholding of sexual creativity from one's sexual partner (low-level passive-aggressiveness)
- achieving orgasm without consideration for pleasuring one's sexual partner
- sexually overt parent-to-child actions such as genital exposure, fondling, or genital penetration
- teacher-to-student flirtations and solicitation of sexual favors
- government officials' sexual harassment of lower-ranking colleagues and/or staff
- businessmen or businesswomen who trade career advancement for sexual favors
- military members and/or their spouses who have sexually oriented relationships with others during times of deployment
- mental health practitioners and/or educators who have sexual relationships with clients or students
- religious leaders who use their positions of power to intimidate and manipulate susceptible victims of their aggression
- depressed and/or mentally disturbed adults who prey sexually on unsuspecting adults or youth
- patrons of major sporting events who participate in organized prostitution in conjunction with the sporting-event-related activities
- internet-based sexual relationships that fail to verify the identities of the online sexual partners
- compulsive sexual practices that dehumanize or depersonalize one's sexual "partner"

- compulsive sexual practices outside the bounds of one's openly declared sexual partnership
- sexual assault and/or rape that may or may not lead to murder
- trafficking of sex slaves for monetary gain.

In addition to seeing and naming sexual violence, individuals must make eradication of sexual violence a priority and outline their personal level and kind of commitment to address it. Also, partnerships with similarly committed members must be developed, publicized, and funded to develop both short- and long-term campaigns and sustainable approaches to reducing the aggression and violence.

We need to feel the pain of sexual violence, and we need to rise up in opposition to it. To do so, we humble ourselves and internalize that by staying silent or by staying small in our vision and efforts, we become a part of the problem. As M. Scott Peck said, advocating the building of community, "It is not impractical to consider seriously changing the rules of the game when the game is clearly killing you."[2]

There is no time to waste. We can start where we are and be open and honest about what we see. Commit to turn the tide, and enlist the support and participation of other awakening souls so that healing can occur in individuals, organizations, and communities and beyond.

Questions for Reflection

1. How has sexual violence affected me? (Consider not only overt physical acts but also exposure to sexual media.)

---

[2] M. Scott Peck, *The Different Drum* (New York: Simon and Schuster, 1987), 18.

2. In what ways has sexual violence (as victim, witness, or perpetrator) affected my sense of self or my ability to be vulnerable to others?

3. How have I acted to bring sexual justice and healing to myself or others in my community? Do my words, actions, thoughts, and beliefs reflect my commitment to ending sexual violence and its damaging effects?

Affirmation

I am open to acknowledging the truth of sexual violence as it has affected my own life and/or others' lives. Moreover, I am committed to bringing justice and healing to those who have been victimized by way of sexual violence.

Day Nine

Question Your Intention before Acting Sexually

This cautionary step is designed to save you lots of heartache. Think of it as the "no regrets" guideline.

By first asking questions of ourselves, we can develop clarity before acting. In fact, the Quakers have a practice called the Clearness Committee. When making key decisions, a Quaker may form a committee of three to five trusted people who spend several hours with them asking them questions. The committee is not permitted to give suggestions, only to ask questions. Thus, by first *giving attention to intention*, a person becomes empowered, which reduces the likelihood of his having to pay for an impulsive or otherwise poor decision for years to come.

Have you heard the phrases "What was I thinking?" and "What were you thinking?" Too often the response is, "I wasn't." And that is the problem.

It may not sound sexy to think of applying critical-thinking skills to our sexual practices, but that is exactly the kind of self-management that demonstrates both wisdom and love. Remember, love is reality-based (truthful), not idealistic or wishful thinking. It shows respect (doesn't violate the other person's well-being and even shows value for the other person's dreams and future potential), is responsible (acts in accordance with both doing no harm and preventing possible harm), and is caring (nurturing, compassionate, kind).

Perhaps it is helpful to consider that eros is not the same as romance. Romance or being romantic occurs when we are in an altered state of seeing only the positive and wanting what we want, now. It is very powerful and serves to guarantee that we will keep the species going, but it does not serve us well when it comes to creating a whole life. Basically it is pleasure seeking at the expense of sensibility. Therefore, preliminary questioning becomes very important. Once one in the throes of romance, questions fly out the window. But consequences do not.

Develop a habit of asking questions. Commit to being clear before you act. This practice of asking questions until you become clear on your motives will serve you well when you surely will be romantic! Consider these "no regrets" questions:

- What will it mean to me if I have sex with this person?
- What will my choice mean to this person if we do have sex?
- Tomorrow, who would I be comfortable telling that this person is my romantic interest?
- To what extent am I ready and trustworthy to make this autonomous/authentic decision?
- How well do I know this person?
- Am I prepared to deal with any potential consequences if I choose to be sexual with this person?
- How anxious am I feeling about this choice?
- Am I willing to wait until I am clear before acting?

Questions for Reflection

1. To what degree have you stopped to ask questions of yourself before making big decisions, both in terms of sexual expression and otherwise?

2. How has your self-questioning, or lack thereof, impacted the course of your life?

3. How do you envision that engaging in consistent self-questioning before making any decisions to act sexually with a partner will affect the outcome of your experiences?

Affirmation

My sexuality is a powerful force. My sexuality is so powerful that I have committed to thinking before, not after, any sexual acts about the potential impact of potential sexual conduct on my life and well-being, along with the life and well-being of my prospective partner.

❧ *Day Ten* ❧

Treat All Persons with Compassion and Respect Regardless of Their Sexual Identity and/ or Sexual Practices

Whole communities, as well as whole cultures, can be guilty of promoting sexual duality, which leads to further isolation and sexual confusion. In contrast, whole communities and whole cultures can evolve in the direction of compassionate sexual worldviews and behavioral-relational patterns.

The Kama Sutra, written centuries ago as a treatise for loving well, is very clear. The writer tells the young traveler that when he enters another person's culture, he is to treat that person and that person's cultural differences with great respect. Similarly, history tells a story of suppression, confusion, oppression, violence, and even disdain for those whose sexual practices deviate from the cultural norms.

State and federal laws tell a similar story of fear, repercussions, repression, and oppression. But more recently, in this era of authenticity, brave people are coming forward and coming out in society to declare their unique sexual identities. Abandoning identities of shame and postures of victimhood, they are standing up to the status quo with its rigid, ironclad ideas of heterosexual superiority. The transition to a sexually positive culture is far from complete. But multiple indicators of irreversible social change suggest progress. Among these are the following:

- A new language is being created. Fifty years ago, homosexuality was considered a psychiatric disorder. Now it is considered one of several sexual identities.
- Sex therapy is becoming mainstream with most marriage and family therapy programs including at least one course in human sexuality.
- Significant advances in the treatment of sexually transmitted diseases have been made. A diagnosis of HIV or AIDS is no longer an automatic death sentence. Both treatment facilities and pharmaceutical companies, as well as nutrition- and wellness-based practices, have become more mainstream.
- Movies, one of our main forms of socially conscious art, are raising social consciousness of issues such as AIDS. For example, both *Dallas Buyers Club* and *Philadelphia* were successful releases in mainstream movie theaters.
- Consciousness is heightened by conflicts regarding the protection of interests of gay, lesbian, bisexual, transgender, or identity-confused individuals.
- Major corporations have made public their positions of respect for persons across the entire spectrum of gender and sexual identity.
- With more and more people coming forward to share their divergent sexual identities and experiences, most, if not all, families are challenged to squarely face the issue of exclusivity vs. inclusivity where sexuality is concerned.

A significant body of research points toward organic causation of sexual orientation. Factors include sex hormone levels while in utero or in some instances development of incongruent or ambiguous sexual genitalia. Furthermore, when persons suffering gender identity confusion tell their stories, it is not unusual for them to relay early memories of recognizing that their sexual orientation differed from that of most of their friends. Similarly, these brave souls tell of encounters wherein they were actively shamed by their parents, siblings, or schoolmates for being "different." As we might expect, at an early age, these individuals began to hide their sexuality, fearing retribution for, not appreciation of, their differences. And even more damning, it seems, is the formation of an identity of shame among the sexually disenfranchised.

It seems appropriate, even an understatement, to say that in response to our growing awareness of how we have treated those with differing sexual identities, we as a society have a responsibility to right the wrongs in our relationships. Whether we feel clear about causation vs. choice is not the primary issue. More importantly, that which is at stake is our acceptance of the obvious diversity of humanity. It is time to acknowledge that we do not have to be threatened by each other, but that we are called to know each other, to embrace each other, and to find ways to live in community. Only when we do this will we ever reach our greatest potential. Conversely, if we do not do this, we will continue to live under an umbrella of real guilt for choosing fear over a spirit of wisdom, empowerment, and love for all.

Questions for Reflection

1. To what degree has your own society and culture related to the diversity of sexual identification?
2. How have you personally felt, over the course of your life so far, about people with types of sexual identification that differ from your own? Have you vilified or befriended them? Have you seen them as being like you or different from you?
3. Has your own sexual identity tended to stay static or to change over the course of your life?

4. Are you comfortable with your own current sexual identity?
    If not, how can you work to build self-acceptance of your
    unique sexual identity?

Affirmation

Everyone has a unique sexual identity. Amid all the world's sexual
diversity, I affirm my own and others' right to love whomever we
choose upon a foundation of adult respect and consent. I also affirm
our common humanity and vow to treat all people with kindness
and compassion regardless of their sexual orientation.

🕊 *Day Eleven* 🕊

As You're Being Your Best You, Remember to Live Your Sexuality in Sync with Your Whole Being

Our humanity transcends but includes sexuality. The two cannot legitimately be disconnected. Knowing this can encourage and instill hope when we're confused or demoralized by our own sexual selves or with that of our friends, our heroes, or even our enemies! At the same time, this integral connection often gives us pause, at a minimum challenging our status quo or tossing us off balance.

It takes self-love and forgiveness to see beyond our sexual behaviors that are either inconsistent with or violate our internal code of conduct. "Who is this person?" we may ask.

Jennine, a young professional attorney, asked this question. Prior to this year, her thirtieth, Jennine lived with behaviors beyond her chronological age. People often commented upon her maturity. But this year something happened that rocked Jennine's world and her family's as well.

Stephen came into Jennine's world. At first the two were committed colleagues who found themselves sharing worldviews and work styles. But beyond that there was an energy that surprised Jennine. At first she dismissed it, thinking it was just nice to finally have a colleague who worked as hard as she and who wanted to make the company a success and build its national reputation. But something happened late one day when the two found themselves alone in the office. Their eyes met. She felt a surge of energy through her body. Looking at Stephen, she realized that he was perspiring. His face had become flushed and his body tense. He was moving toward her. Jennine did not want to stop him.

Later that week, talking with her therapist, Jennine explored her confusion. Up until meeting Stephen, Jennine had tended toward the sensible and normative. Marry the person with whom you can keep order, and keep the economics of family life moving forward. However, Jennine could not forget what had happened between her and Stephen. Nor could she forget her dream in which she was desperately attempting to awaken her husband from a deep sleep, only to have him rise in anger and knock her across the room while screaming, "Let me sleep, you b----!"

Jennine asked her therapist if they could invite her husband to therapy to see if couples work could help awaken a passion between them and to help them learn how to communicate with each other instead of merely coexisting. Sadly, Jennine's husband only came to a couple of therapy sessions. But when he did attend, his posture was one of skepticism and self-protectiveness.

Fast-forward three and a half years. Jennine is now engaged to Stephen, and for the first time in her life Jennine reports that she is happy and hopeful. Longtime friends ask Jennine what has happened to their rational friend who always clicked off strategies with objective clarity and nonemotional entanglements. Now they describe her as softer, more relaxed, fun to be with, both witty and creative, and more alive. Now Jennine's friends find themselves asking questions about their own lives and the choices they have been making. It is in the asking of questions, as Jennine and her friends did, that we invite greater abundance and mystery into our lives.

The reality is that none of us got here without a solid connection to sexuality. Our very belly buttons speak to this connection. They tell us that sometime before we were born, a sperm and egg met and became one, and that unity is us. A new creature, mysterious, multidimensional, carrier of generations of memories perhaps, provides new destinies for many who will be affected by our lives.

Regardless of where we live, we have expectations for what is human and for what is sexual. In addition, we have ideas about what is normal and what is abnormal. Furthermore, when our sexuality fits within the boundaries of our expectations, we tend to feel better about being human. On the other hand, our sexuality can be quite wild and unbridled, defying all our awareness of who we think we are or want to be. We ask, "What makes this so?" Also, we may wonder if and how we can change our relationship with our sexuality so that we are more comfortable, more in control. Or, if we live long enough and don't suppress or repress our sexuality, it may keep showing up, surprising and shocking us, while at the same time leaving us breathless with exhilarating pleasure and ramped-up energy. Consider that it is in this sphere of unbridled, surrendered eros that we find a deep and abiding life force that will not, cannot, be silenced forever.

This is what could be called the learning moment, the space of high potential for transformation. This is so because in the not knowing, in the ambiguity and/or dissonance, we realize that there is something within that is far more powerful than our will, or our learning, or our desire to please others. Simply stated, it is our very life force. It is one form of love that shows up as the desire and will toward pleasure, toward relationship, and toward surrender to something greater than our control and/or our self-protection.

This latter type of learning about the nature of our sexuality has the capacity to awaken us to the fact that life is meant for more than endurance and/or dependability. Life is much like fine aged wine, poured from a chalice onto the bosom or belly of a lover and sucked up with ardent passion. For this reason, may we always remember that in our sexuality, if lived fully, we find our deeper selves!

Questions for Reflection

1. When have you experienced the wild, playful side of eros, either within yourself or within your partner?
2. Do you believe that wild, erotic expression can have a place in life or that is a dangerous force to be put in its place?
3. How can you open to the wildness of eros while maintaining your integrity as a human being in community with others?

Affirmation

The life force that gives sexual life to me—and to everyone on the planet—is a wild and playful force. By developing in wisdom and maturity, I can dance in the storm of this sexual energy, letting it show me more about who I am and who my beloved really is.

Become Aware of the Sexuality-Related Pain of Others

Have you ever known someone for years before learning of some painful experience of a sexual nature that he or she had been carrying while feeling isolated or powerless to move beyond it?

Throughout the years, as either nurse, counselor, or educator, it has been our privilege to sit with people who shared, often for the first time, how they had been hurt deeply by someone who either taunted, harassed, raped, or betrayed them.

Many of these people had immediate family members and a network of friends but had not felt it proper to share their hurtful experiences. They were afraid that they would not be believed, or perhaps they doubted that anyone would take time to help them do anything about what had happened. So they literally suffered in silence until they felt they were in a safe place to share.

To become a "holding place" for someone's pain is both an honorable act as well as a healing practice. But it takes time, intention, and skill. All involved parties will be changed by an experience in which someone who has been hurt deeply in a sexual way can entrust the story to another human being who listens, cares deeply, and responds in a way that communicates respect and appreciation. Such an experience of transparency, vulnerability, and compassion is truly a recipe for meaningful social change.

To help you in this practice, try applying the following guidelines:

1. Remember, any message has multiple layers of meaning, both content and feelings.
2. Listen beyond the details of what a person says for the hidden or embedded messages.
3. Watch for incongruities between what is said and how it is said.
4. Bring your listening presence to others so that the discussion can go beneath the surface.
5. Share enough of your own story to convey that you can handle more than surface chatter.
6. When someone dares to share troublesome or awkward information, sit tight; don't bolt.
7. Don't rescue. Instead, reframe the meaning in your own words to show full understanding.
8. Don't interrogate with questions. Affirm the person's bravery and offer continued support.

A Painful Story

Roxanne came to me after attending a presentation about women and sexuality that was given to a professional women's group. She was struck by the account of the Mayflower Madam, Sydney Barrows, who had created a highly successful escort service in New York City. We talked about the similarities and differences of selling one's body vs. selling one's mind as professors or consultants so often do.

At first the conversation seemed intellectual with Roxanne demonstrating a quick wit and incisive analysis of complex ethical issues. But about an hour into the conversation, Roxanne asked me how I would feel about having access to thousands of files on internet sex clients. To say the least, I was intrigued. How could

I, a professional in the field of human behavior, sexuality, and counseling, reject this gift? But it required risk. My curiosity and intuition won. I invited Roxanne to tell me more.

It seemed that Roxanne was sizing me up, deciding if she was safe to reveal her work as an internet prostitute. She decided that I was safe, and thus as we dialogued, our relationship began. The story of our friendship could be a book in itself, but allow me to share this: During the ensuing months and years, what I learned was that Roxanne used her work to connect with people in pain and to find ways to show them gentleness, respect, and hope. Only deep into the friendship did I begin to see how Roxanne's work mirrored her own pain. Having lived through numerous complicated legal quagmires, as well as her often finding herself in compromising circumstances, she had become a solitary figure within a landscape of so-called privilege. In Roxanne's eyes, I not only knew her, I also accepted her and allowed her to reveal her overwhelming pain. Had I rejected Roxanne because on the surface she is a sex worker, I never would have known her to be an angel of mercy to so many. The loss truly would have been mine.

Questions for Reflection

1. Are you aware of sexuality-related pain that friends, coworkers, or acquaintances may have endured from others, particularly when the offense was a matter of discrimination or oppression toward a member of a minority group?
2. If you are aware of such sexually related suffering, what was your experience of listening to or showing up for this person like? Were you able to bring a spirit of loving-kindness to this person? If so, what effect did your listening have on the other? If not, how do you imagine you might handle the situation differently in the future?

Affirmation

In a world in which so many have endured sexual violence and suffering, I can bring a spirit of open listening and loving-kindness to those who have been hurt, whether someone is openly sharing his or her hurt or I am simply in his or her presence.

Increase Your Sexual Consciousness and You Increase Your Sexual Fulfillment

This may be difficult to picture because you may have grown up in a sexually repressive culture. If this is the case, then you may think of sexual freedom as an escape from the "house rules." If so, this means you stretch the sexual boundaries as much as you dare but try never to get caught. This, of course, is a cat and mouse game, putting you always on the run to avoid being seen. This is anything but free. The consequences are that you live under a shadow of guilt and shame with an increased risk of physical harm, secrecy, isolation, and confusion.

When we learn to repress our sexuality, we don't make it go away; we just marginalize it to the shadows. But being the wild and ever-present force that it is, it will be noticed!

Think of public personas across multiple walks of life and you'll notice examples of this duality. For example, think of former president Bill Clinton, for decades considered the most powerful political figure in the world. And what almost brought him down? His sexuality, repressed, hidden, fragmented, destructive, and yet visible in his charisma. Not until Bill Clinton was publicly shamed and nearly ruined did he reconcile his sexual demons with his deep personal values and his desire to serve something transcendent to himself.

Or in 2016, think of publicly celebrated athletes such as the Stanford world-class swimmer who, while drunk, pulled a young woman behind a shed and brutally sexually assaulted her. Instead of having a winning summer of swimming and fun, his summer was spent in prison. His record and life story changed forever. Or think of the young woman whom he assaulted. While it in no way excuses the young man, her story is also a story of unconsciousness and its accompanying risk—for she must acknowledge that because she drank to the point of unconsciousness, she could not adequately defend herself.

These are painful but very real stories. Unfortunately they make headlines day after day in newspapers, on social media, in professional communications, in police reports, and in counselors' progress notes.

Approximately one in five college coeds can expect to be sexually assaulted during their undergraduate college years. The US military reports of sexual assault are similarly disconcerting. For females returning from war zones who report posttraumatic stress, approximately half of them list sexual assault as the source of trauma.

We see corporate executives with long histories of career success toppled by their sexual indiscretions. For example, Roger Ailes and Bill O'Reilly, formerly of Fox News, were considered among the most powerful influencers of political power, yet both were forced to leave Fox under a cloud of suspicion for reportedly having sexually harassed multiple people over many years. What about the media superstar Bill Cosby, long known for his educational leadership? In 2018, after a trial and mistrial, Cosby was sentenced to three to ten years of imprisonment in Pennsylvania. As of early 2019, Cosby, through his attorney was asserting his innocence and stating that he had no remorse.

Dallas and Atlanta are known as two cities with the highest rates of sex trafficking in the United States. For this to happen, human sexuality must be treated as a commodity that can be traded in the shadows of a free market. Sexual trafficking requires conscious organization, planning, and execution, along with a certain level of secrecy, running, repression, duality, and deliberate cover-ups by people in positions of power. It also requires a climate of support in which it can be bred and grown. In this we are all implicated.

Rooting out sexual evils requires that all of us, starting at the grassroots level, awaken to the reality that our sacred sexuality has been wrested from us while we have slept and while we have sought safety in the confines of our self-protective enclaves.

In August 2016, as the United States and the world geared up for the Olympics, *USA Today* reported on its network investigation "A Blind Eye to Sex Abuse: How USA Gymnastics Protected Coaches over Kids by Failing to Report Allegations of Misconduct." Similar headlines surface across our country and the world, speaking to system-wide avoidance of responsibility for how we manage and/or live our sexuality. While we have embraced unconsciousness, egregious crimes have been committed against humanity. We simply must wake up!

We must name the crime for what it is. It is not "sexuality." It is unconsciousness in the face of rampant hijacking of one of our most sacred birthrights, our capacity to engender new life through the act of coupling.

Think of what it means to "couple": two separate beings come together for the purpose of becoming one to have community and to know and to be known. What could be more precious? But instead of being something that we celebrate and share, sexuality has become guttural (literally as well as figuratively).

Turning this social crisis around is not going to be easy. It will require an enormous army of committed individuals. These individuals must be empowered and conscious. The mission is bold and sacred. It requires being anchored in one's core self. For it is so that at our core, we are consciousness. And once we have awakened to this reality, it becomes more and more difficult to squelch the irrepressible spirit of our being.

It is at this point in our development that we may know sexual fulfillment at all levels of being: mind, body, and spirit.

Questions for Reflection

1. How do you see sexuality being degraded in our popular culture and in our communities?
2. Why do you believe so many people, even people in positions of great power, are able to perpetuate the commodification and debasement of sexuality?
3. What is the relationship between sexual repression and sexual exploitation and violence?

Affirmation

I am awake and aware of sexuality's repression and debasement in my society. As a person committed to my fellow human beings, I will stand up to these forces of sexual violence and ignorance by proclaiming the right of all people to be treated with respect—mentally, physically, and spiritually.

Fiercely Embrace and Guard Your Sexuality; It is Sacred

No kiss is cheap. The first kiss cannot be repeated. Once we've chosen to act sexually, we cannot take the actions back.

Prostitutes know this. If you haven't seen the movie *Pretty Woman*, it's worth seeing. The woman for hire refuses to kiss her client. Think about it!

Kids hookin' up talk about having sexual encounters without any emotional connection. To connect emotionally means to have lost the game. Think about it! Is this a game anyone can really win?

What is being held back? Is it not a misguided attempt to separate ourselves into parts to protect our essence or core self? Somewhere within each of us there is a human spirit, a place that no one else can claim. Oddly enough it is most often in the fray on our intense battlegrounds that we learn intimately of this innate, very intimate aspect of our being.

Victor Frankl, in *Man's Search for Meaning*, describes how the Nazis during World War II stripped the Jewish people of their families and their belongings, even shaving the hair from their bodies, but he discovered that there was one thing the Nazis couldn't take—the human spirit. It has been given to us. It is us. Only we as individuals can surrender it.

Somehow deep within us we know that our sexuality and our spirituality are of one essence. They are mystery. They are power. They are omnipresent. They cannot be bought, even though through every age and across the entire planet they have been sought as if they were for hire. Counterfeits abound. Thus as individuals we must train, much like ninjas. Otherwise, we will be hoodwinked by charlatans masquerading as spiritual and/or sexual masters.

It will take a lifetime of training to become mature sexual ninjas. But during the journey, if we remain both humble and bold, this humble audacity will lead us home to the sacred.

In keeping with the idea that we are warriors in training, we must remember to do the following:

- Seek out ethical, nonexploitive resources to learn more about our sacred sexuality.
- Be willing to hear and benefit from stories of those who have lived well their sexual journeys.
- Practice the art of sacred sexuality as we understand it now—conscious, compassionate, with efficacy, creativity, vulnerability, curiosity, and integrity.
- Receive feedback from our sexual partner and make course corrections as learning occurs.
- Contemplate our development as a practitioner of sacred sexuality, breathing in the delight, owning the style and experiences, and appreciating the contributions of our partner and teacher.
- Allow the beauty and energy engendered by our sexuality to permeate our whole being as attention is drawn to other matters of daily living.
- Honor the day by embracing, once again, the goodness of being who we are, alive, sacred, and sexual.

Questions for Reflection

1. When have I experienced your sexuality as something that is uniquely yours—as a reflection of your deepest self that you can never truly lose?
2. Recall any time(s) when you have not felt or acted with respect for your own sexuality. How did this lack of sexual respect affect your life? How might you handle similar situations or feelings differently in the future?

Affirmation

In the depths of my spirit, I know that I am good. My sexuality, as it reflects my spirit and my unique consciousness, is also good, imbued with the sacredness of life. No one can give me this gift or take it away. My essence and my sexuality are mine—sacred gifts to experience and express in ways that honor my life and the lives of others.

Sexual Wisdom Comes When Sexual Power Is Filtered through the Lens of Love

Long before we have sexual wisdom, we have sexual power. In fact, as discussed on Day One, we are born sexual. But we are also born as infants who require much oversight, training, supervision, and discipline before we ever leave home to make it by ourselves in the world.

A very slim minority of people on our planet are born to mature parents who love each other and who have consciously planned their pregnancies and have structured their two lives to be accessible, caring caretakers, teachers, coaches, advocates, and role models. The rest of us find our way amid varying degrees of chaos, companionship, and perhaps well-meaning but often misguided attempts to be adults. We're a motley crew, a ragtag band of warriors who want the best for ourselves but who hardly know how to get it. We need help. We need wisdom because our sexual energies *will* rise up, and without wisdom, our choices are more likely to divide than to develop.

With this division in mind, let's examine the meaning of several of these core concepts.

First let's look at sexual power. Sexuality is the mysterious force that draws us toward physical experiences of ecstasy, often centered in our genital and/or erotic zones. For many, it is first experienced as auto-arousal through touching one's own body parts to experience pleasurable sensations. Next, during the toddler and preschool years, in the perceived safety and privacy of peer play, pleasure is experienced through mutual touching and play. During these early childhood years, there is an innocence to the child's play. And with nurturing and gentle guidance from adult caregivers, children learn about public and private worlds and how to respect each other's boundaries. But in families and communities where there are many boundary crossings and violations, children learn mixed messages about their bodies, selves, and boundaries. What might be normal rules and norms in one setting or culture might be abnormal in another. But through the mix, children develop maps for how to be and how to relate.

Sexual power in the individually developing person takes on new dimensions and different intensities at each stage of development. And depending upon one's immediate family and community, various types of sexual education occur. Through the interaction of one's developing experiences and education, individuals express their sexual power. It could be in music, sports, group participation, dating, fashion, secret hook-ups, social media, or other means of expression.

At the same time, family communication and educational systems attempt to shape youth in prescribed ways. Core values are imparted by parents, in sex education classes, or from religious institutions. Judgment and perhaps enforcement may be part of the messages. Youth are often cautioned with consequences and fear of repercussions. And youth observe, discuss, and decide to what extent and in what manner they will conform. So begins the development of one's level of conscious sexuality. With increased amounts of unsupervised time, youths will experiment with their sexual power.

During the time when bodies and hormone levels are changing, adolescents are forming their identities. Perhaps at no other time during one's life span is it more important to have validation and confirmation of one's inherent worth. By inherent, we mean inborn, natural, even God-given worth and value. If this affirmation is present, then this nurturing, meaningful guidance, and encouragement can prepare the young person to launch her exit from home, to prepare for meaningful work, and to consider with whom she will partner. As the young person builds a lifetime community of two, she is free to contribute to the next generation of people, as well as to the next generation of socioeconomic organizations. But if this meaningful feedback is trivialized or not viewed as significant, the young person emerges wounded, confused, destined through trial and error to find her own way and to create paths where she hits dead ends or where there are no clear cues for how to proceed. And because sexuality or sexual power is one of the most potent aspects of being human, it will be included in the mix of significant experiences.

Back to our definitions:

Power is the ability to act with significant influence to affect the processes and/or outcomes of the action.

Sexual power is the ability to affect one's own or another's quality, awareness, and experience of sexuality. Some questions to consider when understanding where and how you have sexual power are as follows:

- Do I use my sexuality to punish my partner by withholding what I know he or she most desires?
- Do I use, or have I ever used, sexuality to reward my partner to get what I want in the relationship?
- Have I ever considered that my motivation for having sex was to maintain a place in my partner's life and to be needed?
- When I choose to have sex, is my desire coming from my need or my desire to receive pleasure and give pleasure?

Wisdom is the application of reason and intuition to one's decisions and actions in a manner that achieves outcomes that either improve or sustain a high quality of life or well-being.

People generally considered to be wise consistently do the following:

- Act with kindness and respect toward all beings.
- Conduct themselves with honor, bringing dignity and just rewards to those within their spheres of influence.
- Apply themselves diligently, with conviction and purpose, to admirable goals.
- Study to show themselves to be responsible, generative contributors to the whole community.
- Communicate with everyone from their genuine, authentic selves.
- Fulfill their personal and societal commitments.
- Make decisions with courage, speaking with vision, authority, clarity, precision, and hope.
- Include everyone in their commitment to kindness, justice, and equality for all human beings.
- Love others in ways that are responsible, authentic, and compassionate.

Love is! And because of love, as the unseen order of things, we can relax in terms of knowing that when we do not know, there is still the One who does know. While our lives depend upon this love, it defies any complete knowing, controlling, or mastery. We can know this: love is life-affirming, life-supporting, and good.

This includes our sexuality in all its paradoxical nature, fierce, wild, burning, and unrelenting yet blissful, beautiful, and whole! Sexuality experienced at this level takes our breath away as we sit or lie in oneness, eyes wide open, looking into the depths of each other: kind and gentle, spent, embracing, so full of hope that it can hardly be contained. While only moments before our passion surged, now tears of compassion emerge, and, as lovers, we simply are. Pure joy and awe!

Note: This image of mature alchemical sexuality is a far cry from sexual violence, promiscuity, cheap thrills, or pornography.

Questions for Reflection

1. Have you every connected the qualities of sexual power with wisdom and love before today?
2. Can you think of any times when you have experienced or witnessed an expression of sexual power that was connected to wisdom and love?
3. Imagine your own experiences of sexual power. Did you experience your sexual power in connection to love or to something else?
4. How has your experience of sexual power impacted the course of your life?

Affirmation

As a sexual being, I have enormous power to do good or to do harm—to myself and others. It is only when I begin and remain in a spirit of love that my sexual power becomes something even greater—real sexual wisdom.

Acknowledge that Your Sexual Worldview Frames Your Sexual Experiences

Everybody has a worldview—everybody. Generally speaking, our worldview is the lens through which we see life. Years ago I knew a man who, whenever you would encounter him and ask how he was, would say, "Hanging in there. Doing the best I can." After a while it occurred to me that those statements were really a reflection of his worldview, which was "Life is a struggle." As I listened more carefully, it became clear that no matter what occurred in his life, good or bad, he saw it through the lens of difficulty and struggle. Just as a worldview frames all your experiences and the meaning you give them, your sexual worldview does the same. Craft it carefully.

One of the most sexually active people I've ever known was a woman who weighed over 300 pounds and boasted in person about having had sex with about 150 people. Watching this woman at work was like watching poetry in motion. You could be in a room filled with about 5 men and 25 women, and she'd leave the party with the man or men of her choice. This woman was winsome. She knew this about herself and made it her mission to live up to her reputation and her self-concept. In short, this woman's sexual worldview was very simple: "My sexuality is what I choose it to be. If I see myself as sexy and project this image, you are within my grasp. I reel you in with my strategy of sexual seduction. I am the pussycat, and you are my mouse."

This woman needed no props, no diets, no setup. She was clear about how she saw sex and the male–female relationship, and it worked for her in terms of seduction and snaring men. Where her worldview stopped, so did her relationships. You see, she saw sexuality and sexual relationships as a game. The goal was to snare the date, over and over again. Sexuality was about "winning." Never did she allow herself to risk shifting to a worldview that frames sexuality and intimacy as more complex and difficult to master.

Or there is the male celebrity within a certain organization. He knows he's considered the most handsome man about town and plays to this image of himself. As he enters a room, heads turn his way and both men and women begin to circle about. There is male joking and jostling about while the women stand back, laughing and watching. Eventually men fall off into various spots and our focal male makes his way to the bevy of women gathered about. Subtly but distinctly his attention becomes more focused on one particular woman, always a pretty woman by the culture's standards. This is the power couple. They carry themselves in accord with their top positions in the hierarchy.

In our second example, there isn't an overt mention of sexuality, but there are the cues of exclusivity, which are taken to mean "hands off" to all the other players. In addition, there are the brief moments of contact, the prized looks, the comments, and the acknowledgments of seeing and being seen. It is the sexual dance. Even to participate, to breathe the same air and share the same space, is considered an honor. It is a taste of the excitement that all imagine happens when the privileged couple is alone. It is another worldview that suggests that sexuality is about attractiveness and power, about being chosen, and about a secret life behind a veil.

We all have a worldview. For many adults, their worldview remains held by their family of origin. For example, some cultures suggest that men pursue the women and that women respond. If women in such a culture are too assertive or aggressive, they are seen to be crossing expected boundaries and are frowned upon. Or, in the same culture, if a man exhibits too many behaviors that are typically attributed to women, he is considered too effeminate and most likely will be the butt of jokes. For the women in this culture, being engaged or married by a predetermined age is very important. Men in this culture are afforded more leeway in terms of when they marry, but if they haven't married by a certain age, questions about their masculinity and sexual orientation surface. Often family members exert significant pressure upon them to find a good woman and settle down. Prejudice can take various forms. For example, men who choose to be ministers may find it difficult to obtain a pulpit position if not married. In this culture, one either shifts worldviews or is expected to comply rather than to create out of his or her own eros. We could say that in this culture, eros is feared and repressed, only to surface in innuendos, advertisements, and jokes.

As you reflect upon these examples, consider the worldview that you have inherited. Next, think about ways in which you may have departed from your original worldview or have begun to question the status quo.

Certain types of experiences can influence our worldview. This can be something like travel to another part of the world, particularly if it is for longer than a standard vacation.

Military members and their families, if stationed in other countries or on other continents, often find themselves learning to see things in new and different ways. Or members of a certain religious group may find that when they get to know and be friends with people from other faith-based systems, they share many of the same ideals and life goals.

So it is in stepping out from the familiar, in asking questions, and in learning to value and appreciate other points of view that we begin to adopt a bigger, more inclusive point of view.

Another significant type of influencer upon our worldview is our educational experiences. For example, when we learn critical thinking and creative thinking skills, we are encouraged to think outside the box, to challenge old assumptions/teachings that were handed down to us, to find new ways to see old problems, to generate solutions together, and to hold the ambiguity long enough to see where the mystery may take us.

Beyond the power of experiences, travel, and education to shift our worldview is another type of influencer that is quite paradoxical in nature: unrelenting and seemingly irreversible pain and loss, the kind that happens when one is betrayed by a trusted intimate sexual partner. At first there's the shock, the disbelief, and then comes the bargaining as we attempt to restore what we had before. But when that doesn't happen, we find ourselves in new territory. Some of our friends no longer show up. We feel lost without an anchor. Old habits no longer are options for soothing. We find ourselves anxious without the usual addictions that we've used to hide our fears and insecurities. We may replace the old habits with new ones that work for a while, but we still yearn to go back. Only there is no back to go to. Thus, we are sent into the chaos of a relationship wilderness zone. If we can manage the anxiety and avoid being rescued, we stand a good chance of learning a new way through. We soften our viewpoints toward things and people who are new and different. We experiment with new ideas, new approaches, new vantage points. Our edges aren't as sharp; our retorts, less frequent. We make space for dialogue instead of launching quick defenses. We are birthing new potentials in our new lives.

Consider the following two groups of people:

Group A

Small, homogenous group of adults who have lived most of their adult lives in predictable circumstances. They are college-educated small families with good jobs who take annual vacations together on worship together on Sundays. Most live into their seventies or eighties. None have been divorced, and no one spouse has come out of the closet as LGBTQ.

Group B

Large, open group of adults, none of whom have lived in the local community more than two years. Several couples are in their second marriages. Two of the women have recently shared that they are in contentious trials with their ex-spouses, and in both cases, the spouse has been charged with sexual violence in the home, one with incest with a stepdaughter.

Questions for Reflection

1. How do you think sexual worldviews impacted the people in group A and group B? Specifically, how do you think these people's worldviews impacted their sexual experiences?

2. Now, consider these two groups in terms of your own sexual worldview, both the one you grew up with and the one you now live out. How do you respond mentally and emotionally to these groups of people based on your sexual worldview?

3. Now consider how your own sexual worldview has impacted your personal sexual and relationship choices. Has your sexual worldview brought you joy and satisfaction or pain and suffering—or perhaps some combination of the two?

4. Can you identify any aspects of your sexual worldview that you would like to change for the benefit of your own health, happiness, and well-being?

Affirmation

My sexual worldview is a powerful determiner of the nature of my sexual choices and experiences throughout my life. Because of this power, I will adopt a sexual worldview that includes more _________________ and _____________________ in order to increase the joy, pleasure, and integrity of my both myself and any partner with whom I choose to share a sexual relationship.

Sexuality is hard to deal with, but can you really imagine a world without it? There would be no orgasms, no need for flirtations, no enticement to make babies—well, scratch that last point, but you have to admit that carrying around another creature inside your belly while it kicks, brings on bouts of nausea, and usually results in at least a little tear when it bursts out, often with a loud announcement cry, is not a typical advertisement script!

Sexuality is a paradox because it exists along a continuum. At one end, it is sheer maddening darkness, and at the other end, it is all blissful sighs and sensations. Where people get into trouble is in trying to ignore, suppress, or repress behavior at one end of the spectrum while embracing the opposite end. Another futile approach is to soften or modulate sexuality so that it gets the job of sexual release and/or procreation done but without much ado about anything. Any of these approaches is just partial truth, which of course we know is a devilish trick. You know the old adage about tricking the fools into thinking it's a "this" when we know it's both: a this and a that. By the time they awaken to discover the truth, we'll be long gone.

As each of us has coursed our way down the path toward an active sex life, we have probably heard all sorts of messages about sexuality, and we will have identified ourselves with one or more camps. If we have stayed close to home, have kept our lives simple, and haven't asked too many questions, then perhaps we have managed to avoid any major confrontations with our sexual paradigm/worldview. On the other hand, if we've experienced sexuality in some degree of variance from what we were taught it was, our eyes have been opened. There is no going back to the either–or thinking. It's no longer possible to make sexuality a this or a that. It is both–and.

It is at this point of conscious awakening that we must confront the disparities, the incongruities, the positives, and the negatives. But how do we do that? We must figure out what it means to embrace the paradox.

Years ago, Wayne Dyer spoke about how to deal with tough issues in our lives. He likened them to snakes, and his motto was "Embrace the snake." This metaphor seems to fit with how we deal with both sexual pain or trauma and sexual fulfillment and joy.

Dyer went on to say that if a snake were on the stage where he was standing, he couldn't deal adequately with the snake if he avoided it or ran to the opposite end of the stage. Quite the opposite. Dyer asserted, "I would have to walk over to the snake, pick it up, and take it out. I would have to embrace the snake." Remember that snakes historically have represented not just danger but also wisdom and sacredness in stories about overcoming the toughest of situations that we encounter!

To us, this is how it is with sexuality; it is sacred and scary! If we think back to our discussion about what it means to be human, we see that we are both ego and spirit, creation and creator. This awareness can help us as we think about our sexuality. Think of it this way: We are made with a core, a nonphysical essence or spirit. It is a good gift to us. We also have an ego, or form, or body in which we carry our core/essence. We might call it our body/mind/heart or our personality template in our body. Whatever we call this, by adulthood we will have struggled inwardly with opposing attributes:

pride and humility, self-aggrandizement and gratitude, compulsion and creativity.

And no matter where we live on the planet, one of the arenas in which we experience this struggle is the sexual arena. We must work out our conflict between being ruled by our sexuality or surrendering our sexuality to a purpose higher or deeper than ourselves.

The struggle is real and cannot be avoided. Even if we have never committed what might be called a "sexual sin," we must at some point in our lives, and in some way, either own or disown our full sexuality.

To embrace the paradox of our sexuality means that we own our sexuality, receive it as a gift and as a responsibility, and live it out in submission to what is most congruent with our inner core or higher self/spirit.

This act of "embracing" is a whole process that consists of multiple acts experienced over a period of time. In addition, it will rarely, if ever, happen as a straight line with one positive choice after another. A significant piece of the embracing will be the struggle, the ups and the downs, and the almost knockouts, followed by the surges of brilliant and compassionate power. It takes time. It is humbling, but if we persist and if we don't deny our reality, then in the end, embracing the paradox of our sexuality replenishes our bodies and renews our souls.

And so it is that we learn to embrace the snake of sexual power, growing in wisdom and love.

Questions for Reflection

1. To what extent do you feel that you have owned or disowned the power of your sexuality over the course of your life?

2. Why do you think it is important to acknowledge the wild and dangerous aspect of your sexual nature?
3. How do you imagine that owning the paradoxical nature of your sexuality could impact your ability to live a whole, healthy, happy life?

Affirmation

My sexuality is a paradoxical power, bringing the potential for both chaos and destruction, along with the potential for deep, abiding sensuality and pleasure. Because of this dual nature of my sexual power, I must work continuously to surrender my sexual choices to the principles and priorities that include me but transcend me as an individual. I intend to grow in my ability to make sexual choices that bring honor to the power of my sexual nature and to the sacredness of my partner as well.

Day Eighteen

Refuse to Wear the Mantle of Sexual Shame

"Shame on you!" Have you ever heard this statement? If so, you know some of what it means to be shamed. Unfortunately, this is how some parents or caregivers try to parent. But it is not wise to use shaming to teach discipline.

What we have discovered in our study of human development is that very early in our lives we learn to think of ourselves as good boys and girls or as bad boys and girls. We learn this through our explorations and from our caregivers' responses to these explorations. If we are taught that we are a bad self, we create a shame-based way of seeing ourselves. Contrast this with learning that we are good, which leads to a sense of potency and effectiveness. We connect being ourselves with a confidence to step out into our world.

Through all our complex interactions based upon our template and that of our surroundings, we come to think and say to ourselves, "I am bad" or "I am good." The name for "I am bad" is *shame.* I define myself as bad. If I think I am bad, I become more and more timid. I hold myself back, doubting that it's okay to venture out, or thinking that if I do, I'll screw up. Because all repressed energy begs expression, we can become aggressive with our sexuality. Whether we receive the affirmation of either "good" or "bad," both are distortions of who we really are at the core. Neither is an affirmation of our true self.

On the other hand, if the feedback and caregiving that we receive teaches us to think that certain things or choices are bad but that we are worthwhile and capable of learning a better way, then we tend to develop along a different path that leads to more self-trust and to autonomous, self-initiating types of choices and behaviors.

How does all this early development connect to our sexuality?

When a child is young, he or she is going to engage in sexual play. This is a normal part of development—to experience bodily pleasure and to satisfy curiosity. And children will often explore sexually with whatever gender their playmates are, typically the same sex.

Now let's say a parent or caregiver discovers two children engaged in sexual play. In one case, the parent may have a strong reaction of shock or horror, telling the children to stop immediately because the behavior is wrong or "not nice." This adult may even say he or she is going to tell the visiting child's parent. It would follow then that the children would feel shame and embarrassment and be timid about initiating learning about sexuality in the future. They've been shut down.

Take the same children in the same situation, but apply a different adult reaction. This time the parent or caregiver stays calm, perhaps says something like, "Hey, guys, I'd like you to put your clothes back on and come out to see [what I'm baking, or what the dog is doing, or a program you might enjoy watching, or a game you can play]." Later, the parent could talk with his or her child, affirming how touching can make the body feel good, the importance of taking care of and respecting the private body parts, and respecting the other child's body parts. Allowing the child to ask questions in a nonjudgmental environment goes a long way toward affirming the goodness of the child's sexuality and preventing shame around his or her natural exploration from setting in.

When we are children, the role of our caregivers is critical to how we develop a view of our sexuality. We must have some sense of hope, and this comes from having those around us in whom we can trust. Not everyone we depend upon will be trustworthy. Some of our caretakers let us down, betray us, and hurt us. But if we have at least one person who loves us and is trustworthy, it can give us hope. For some of us as adults, we may have learned to doubt not only ourselves but also that anyone can help us. If this is our story but we are still willing to learn and give life a chance, then even in adulthood we can change our story. We do not have to let doubt and shame win! We can find a way to live with honor, integrity, and creativity. But to do so, we must take some risks. Perhaps we must create some chaos along the way. Even so, there is still hope.

In addition, we must see how much we trust or mistrust ourselves. To do this, we must check our self-talk. What are the messages that we tell ourselves in terms of who we are and how well we think of ourselves? Would we treat someone else as badly or as well as we treat ourselves? What do we really believe about ourselves, because, as much as anything else, this will determine how we live our lives.

Instead of shaming ourselves, we must call our own hand. To do so, we must ask if we are being self-destructive. We may need someone wiser than we to help us look at our story to determine if we are shame-based. If so, we need to carefully select a wise friend or a professional counselor/coach/mentor to help us look at ourselves and conduct an honest self-inventory.

Questions for Reflection

1. Do I realize that shame applies to an action but is not a definition of my whole personhood? For example, I can do a shameful act, meaning I can act without healthy regard

for myself and/or for another, but to act shamefully does not make me a shameful person.

2. When I feel shame, do I recognize what is happening? Will I allow myself to stop and investigate the message of my feelings and then walk myself through the situation proactively rather than reactively, knowing that as long as I'm alive, I have another opportunity to act from a place of trustworthiness and integrity?

3. When I fall down, do I routinely allow my negative self-talk and habits to keep pulling me down, or do I have a tool bag of helpful, healthy things I know to do that I draw from instead?

4. Do I isolate, which is the position of shame (picture shame as pulling you into a ball like a fetus in the mother's womb), or do I make a point of connecting with at least one healthy person? For example, I may be alone in my house, but if I have one piece of working technology, I can find a channel or source of a positive message, basically 24/7. Shame feeds on isolation and self-defeatism.

5. If I know that I have a shame-based identity and life pattern, do I build up a store of resources and keep them handy for when the old habits arise? For example, if I soothe myself with pornography, do I destroy the pornography and replace it with a stock of artwork, music, short inspirational writings about healthy relationships, or other uplifting resources? Do I include in my emergency kit things such as yoga exercises, breathing instructions, music libraries, or other self-discipline/self-affirming tools?

6. Do I create an environment that is "anti-shame"— congruent and self-affirming? My personal space may only be something like 6' × 6', but if it's my space, I can infuse it with beauty, such as an uplifting quote on the mirror, a rug that is made from scraps of colors that I like and have woven, a chair cushion that includes my favorite photo of a pet, a

throw for when I'm chilly, and a sense of organization—dishes clean, bed made, magazines and books organized.

Shame grows where kindness, respect, dialogue, and creativity are nonexistent or have been silenced. But the truth is and always has been that each of us comes into this world with inherent worth and tremendous value. This is a given. We all begin in the mind of the same Source that transcends any and all circumstances. So, no matter the circumstances of our conception or of our physical existence, we have a home base, a soul that is nonphysical/spirit. We are, at our core, of great value. Just as Victor Frankl learned, we can learn that no one and nothing can take away our human spirit!

Affirmations

I am of great value. I give thanks to my Creator for my life.

This day is good because I live. I will leave this day better than I found it.

With each breath, I demonstrate courage. Today I breathe deeply with hope and dedication to make a positive difference wherever I go.

I am good. I use my sexuality for good, being intentional, disciplined, and loving.

I am sexual. My sexuality is one part of my being creative. With my sexual being, I will create only that which is honorable, joyful, and life-giving.

Let Go of Memories of Experiences in which You Feel Helpless

You do not have to be bound by past sexual experiences. Instead, you can learn to let go of memories of experiences that render you any degree of helpless.

If we consider things realistically, then we must admit that none of us know for sure how long we humans have been on this planet. Nor do we know exactly how our current codes of sexuality have evolved. But we do have stories. Taken collectively, these stories comprise history. It is within the domain of history where the problem lies.

History is a story told largely through a masculine, cultural lens. This worldview or paradigm for ascribing normalcy to sexuality based upon gender impacts both men and women, often prescribing roles that don't fit the person(s). Today, scientists and practitioners suggest that gender seems to exist along a continuum rather than existing as two distinctly different categories of being. But the powerful mantel of sexual norms overshadows many of us, so we find ourselves affected by, if not enslaved by, old, prescriptive, and disempowering belief systems. We must let go of our old mind-sets if we are to connect with new hope and potential. Examples of this universally freeing process of *emptiness* or *letting go* are seen throughout history. Following are some examples from which we can learn to stop, see ourselves, forgive our lesser choices, and open ourselves to restorative, even transformative, relationships.

The book of Solomon, or Song of Songs as it is called, tells the story of King Solomon, often called the wisest of men. As is told in the Hebrew Bible (1 Kings 11:1–40), this man Solomon strayed from his relationship with God and from his covenant with his wife / young lover. He wandered for years, taking many wives, only later to, as the book of Ecclesiastes describes, return to his original awareness that life's truest meaning comes in knowing and being faithful to one's Creator, whose purpose and presence transcends any human transgression. And so it is that today each of us may wander. We may act with ignorance, selfishness, or malice toward others, but it is possible for us to make transformative changes that restore us to our original state of intimacy and unconditional acceptance and authenticity. This message of *change* offers each of us hope. But we must accept and act upon its availability in order to realize its freedoms.

Anthropologist Riane Eisler, in *Sacred Pleasure*, describes how our patriarchal control-and-dominate culture actually came about as people migrated away from fertile land with abundant food supplies and as competition overtook partnership as the normative way of being in community. According to Eisler, people previously lived together with collaboration and equality and with both femininity and masculinity being valued and integrated into daily living. Thus, drawing from Eisler's work, we might say that our deepest roots are in equality, not domination. It is up to us to let go of external hierarchal models and replace them with models of power that celebrate our core unity while embracing our individual uniqueness.

When we choose helplessness, we diminish ourselves and the contributions that we are here to make.

Furthermore, we render ourselves as less than we are. Helplessness is a kissing cousin to shame because it assumes that we have lost before we even begin to consider what creative options might be open to us.

When we retell a story of the past in which we were the underdog or in which we failed to achieve our goal as if such a thing defines who we are, we create a self-fulfilling prophecy, meaning that we end up creating the very things we fear. Thus new, more satisfying outcomes can only be achieved when we extricate ourselves from our past experiences. This means that we must, in our mind's eye, step back and reexperience the old experience/memory, but this time change the dynamics to allow for either new actions or new meaning. To put it differently, we must question the meaning we have ascribed to the past experience. And, maybe even more importantly, we must give ourselves permission to say, "This is not me. Yes, I did that then. But now I have learned [x, y, z], and I am no longer willing to do that or be there. Today I am here, right now, and I choose [a, b, c]." When we do this, we acknowledge that we are open, learning, growing systems capable of continuous renewal. Yay us!

Neither of us authors expect or ask that you rewrite your whole history or culture in thirty-one days, but we absolutely do believe that as you choose to get in touch with the pressures and expectations that do exist, you will be better prepared to think and act for yourself in terms of your sexual freedoms and/or constraints.

Here are several concrete things you can do to wrest your sexual decision-making from the jaws of external or internal predetermined, discriminatory moral directives:

1. Step back from prescribed musts or shoulds so you can see these matters more clearly in terms of their intended outcomes and underlying assumptions.

2. When you have been on the receiving end of harsh, disrespectful, hurtful sexual choices and/or behaviors, declare your intention *not* to be defined by someone else's uncaring and/or harmful way of being.

3. When you have been on the offending end of harsh, disrespectful, hurtful sexual choices and/or behaviors,

declare your intention to no longer act in ways that are noncaring and/or hurtful.

4. Remember that memories are reconstructions of what happened. They embody what we recall as having happened and include filters for how to make sense of what happened. This awareness provides space in which to reframe or rewrite how we relate to our past experiences.

Questions for Reflection

1. When have you experienced musts or shoulds related to the expression of your sexuality? How do you believe these cultural or societal expectations affected the decisions you made related to your sexual behavior?
2. If you have ever been on the receiving end of harsh, disrespectful, or hurtful sexual choices, how do the offending person's actions affect your self-definition?
3. Have you ever inflicted harsh, disrespectful, or hurtful sexual choices or behaviors onto another person? If so, have you faced the consequences of your choices and moved forward with your life in a space of self-honesty and self-forgiveness?

Affirmation

I am not my experiences. As a free, unique individual, I choose to put my experiences into context—to learn from the experiences but not be defined by them. Today I am free to change any relationship patterns that keep me smaller than I am meant to be.

Communicate Sexual Messages Forthrightly by Saying What You Want in Appropriate and Effective Ways while Conveying Understanding of and Insight into Potential Outcomes

A person may participate in intense sexual experiences but become timid, even fearful, when attempting to bring about change in his or her sexual relationship. Our sexual communications can become clearer and more effective.

Here are some examples of sexual messages that beg to be communicated:

- What is pleasurable, preferred, liked
- Embarrassment about body changes due to aging, health, surgery
- Body image issues around penis size, breast size, cellulite, hip size, stomach size
- Sensitive areas on one's body
- When something is painful or uncomfortable
- When one does not want to have sexual intercourse
- When one does want to have sexual intercourse
- When sexual play has more appeal that sexual intercourse
- Sharing sexual fantasies and wanting to act on these

- Not feeling very attractive or sexual
- Not feeling attracted to one's partner at the moment
- Partner's body odor, breath, etc., is unappealing
- Discussion of birth control with new partner
- Telling a new partner of a sexually transmitted disease
- Not enjoying a partner's kissing style
- Asking questions of a new partner about sexually transmitted diseases

As we have stated before, *love*, according to Erich Fromm, has four main components: knowledge, care, respect, and responsibility. We would add a fifth, truth. The cornerstone of civility is not politeness. The cornerstone of civility is truth. So then what if we could learn to *speak truth in love* when we needed to open the dialogue and deliver our sexual messages? If we're honest, this would require learning and practice for every one of us.

If your perception is that you have a significant role in creating a high-quality, mutually gratifying, sex-positive relationship, then you want to respond to you partner in ways that are encouraging to him or her but that also speak the truth about what you would like to see different—to make each of your experiences more wonderful!

Consider questions such as "Do I want to know the other person? Do I want to be known by the other person?" Communication that fosters *knowing* the other and *being known* by the other requires us to have courage and vulnerability. Without these traits, no relationship can thrive or be truly life-giving. We must be willing to boldly but kindly speak our truth with *humble audacity.* And we especially must be willing to show up and be vulnerable, risking the very things we wished to avoid by remaining silent: judgment and rejection. Think about the alternative. If we say nothing and we continue as we have been, we risk hurting our partner (e.g., by not disclosing an STD), risk harming ourselves by not inquiring about our partner's health history, or continue to have a less-than sexual relationship. In our culture, we see countless other consequences of poor communication such as unwanted pregnancies, contracting STDs, or perhaps engaging in a sexual relationship that one doesn't want.

Questions for Reflection

1. When communicating with your partner, are you clear about the truth you want to convey as to your purpose for bringing up a particular topic? Are you clear about the need within you that you are trying to get met? Is your need or want legitimate, fair, respectful, and good?

2. How well do you tend to know your sexual partner? Can you see and name his or her areas of emotional and personal sensitivity or insecurity without judgment? Do you have empathy for him or her? In other words, are you able to put yourself in his or her shoes, to truly see things through her or his eyes in such a way that you can feel what it's like to be your partner in this particular situation?

3. Do you care enough about your partner so that you want to choose your words carefully and not intentionally inflict hurt on him or her? By doing this, you demonstrate compassion. Compassion is the ability to be "with" the other person, an understanding that you, too, can imagine what it's like to be in your partner's position or have his or her experience.

4. How aware are you of your influence on your partner? Do you understand that your words carry a punch? Words matter. Are you a truth-teller? Do you see your partner as who he or she and not as who you want him or her to be?

5. Ask yourself, "To what extent do I feel responsible for the quality of our sexual relationship?"

Affirmation

My communications with my partner are powerful and influence the quality of our lives, both as individuals and as a couple. When I communicate from a place of clear intentions with humility, combined with boldness and deep care and love for my partner, we are better equipped for sharing life experiences—including and transcending our sexual relationship—that build not only enhanced pleasure but also enhanced joy and well-being in both our lives.

Take Part in Creating New, More Effective Approaches to Sexually Troubling Social Issues

While becoming a social advocate for healthy sexuality may seem daunting or may send you running for fear that you will be stretched way beyond your comfort zone, this is not what we have in mind. However, we do believe that we are here on planet Earth to make a difference—and many differences need to be made when it comes to sexuality.

Allow us to list just a few of the social injustices that occur every day with regard to sexuality:

- Children are taken by social services from their homes because either a parent or sibling has sexually assaulted them.
- Many counties within most states now report that human sex trafficking is an ever-present concern of the local family court services.
- Young, naive teens are sexually assaulted while on dates with someone they have trusted.
- Female military members often report that the major source of their PTSD has been sexual violations from their own peers or supervisors.
- Too many suicides occur because individuals have been bullied or shamed for their sexual identity or preferences.

- Countless numbers of employees cower sexually to bosses who hold power over them for job stability or advancement.
- Unwanted babies are conceived and born because of faulty or scant information or contraceptive resources, as well as ambiguous definitions of responsibility for safe sex.

To make a real, measurable difference in people's lives, you can consider several time-tested methods. Read the following list and choose a place to start. Then write your commitment and, using your phone calendar, mark dates at one-week, two-week, and one-month intervals from today as checkpoints on your progress.

1. Choose one sexually challenging issue to focus on right now. The issue I choose is _______________________.
2. Go online and research the issue, identifying reasons, impacts, number of people affected, underlying dynamics and arguments, funding issues, people of influence who share your concern, and people and offices that might make a difference, among other things.
3. Meditate upon what bothers you most about the issue. Draw inspiration for some wisdom from writing, music, art, and nature—examples that resonate. Allow your inner eyes to draw you to images of change.
4. Connect in your head, your heart, and your body with the pain of the issue. Ask, "What can I do?"
5. Here are some examples of what people choose to do. There are many more, but let these stimulate your ideas:
   a. Confront a person you are dating.
   b. Apologize if you have contributed to the issue in a way that has hurt someone.
   c. Talk with a friend, and together decide how to make a difference.

    d. Go to a person with organizational position power who can inform you of resources. Examples: school counselor, school security officer, employee communications liaison, the sexual assault prevention or report officer on a military base, religious leaders.

    e. Take a course online or locally that addresses intimacy, communications, personal power, applications of faith and principles, etc.

    f. Join an organization that provides regularly occurring opportunities for group dialogue.

    g. Become a student of social change, and find ways to interject new, more comprehensive solutions to social needs that require time, money, changes in policy, and more.

    h. Be available to friends who share that they are experiencing one of these issues.

Remember that social change occurs when small groups of people commit and then keep their commitments to reach out in love and care to those who have real-time needs. And never, ever forget that underlying group action, there are the choices and actions of individuals who are living by the following motto: *If it is to be, it is up to me!*

Questions for Reflection

1. Do you think of yourself as having the power to make a difference in the sexual health and well-being of not just yourself but also your community and/or society at large?

2. To what degree have you read, listened to, and learned about sexual issues that are hurting your society?

3. What aspects of sexual health in society concern you most, and why?

4. What actions, big or small, can you take in your own life to learn more and to positively impact the sexual health issue that concerns you most deeply?

Affirmation

In my own unique way, I am committed to becoming more knowledgeable about issues related to sexual health in society and to reaching out as an agent of compassion, healing, and change in relation to these issues.

Day Twenty-Two

Pay Attention to Your Self-Talk

Consider your self-talk. This is one of your most important tools when it comes to knowing yourself. The things you say to yourself when you are alone or are being honest with yourself are the clues to knowing yourself. These words, these messages, indicate to you the extent to which you are empowered. Trust yourself; believe that the choice is truly yours. Your self-talk tells you of the consequences that you imagine given different choices. Based upon what you say to yourself and how you hear what you say, you will make a choice. An interesting study done awhile back suggests that people who talk to themselves using their name, for example, "Mary, you can talk to him about this," were more likely to have positive outcomes than people whose self-talk goes like "I can talk to him about this." Just a little tip.

A number of things factor into your decision, but one is the extent to which you tell yourself that your welfare is dependent upon the response of your boyfriend, your girlfriend, your mother, or anyone else. Think about it. When we give someone else the option of deciding whether or not we are okay, we have given away our power. Before we can own our sexuality, we must learn that our self-worth and our being is not dependent upon anyone else. It is a given that we are born with. And while it is natural that, as infants and small children, our welfare is dependent upon other people, as we grow into adulthood, it is important for us to find ways to reclaim our power.

Just in case you are in abusive and/or oppressive circumstances, it is important to know that while other people may take away all your external freedoms, they can never claim your soul, your human spirit. That is yours. It goes with you wherever you go, including when your soul exits your body to return to our source. So, when your anxiety tends to rise, remember this: *I am not my experiences. My essence and worth are not dependent upon anyone else. They are given to me and are mine to own, to appreciate, and to develop.*

Several years ago, after much work on her self-talk and self-affirmation, a woman gave me a plaque to put in my office so that everyone could read it. It said, "I am enough." To this day I believe that this statement reflected the new, more intimate relationship she had developed with herself. She realized a truth for all of us. Just as our words to others influence the quality of our relationships with them, so the words to ourselves impact our relationship with ourselves.

As we become more and more intimate with our core / inner selves, we trust that we are here by design with a unique purpose and mission that was written long before we were born. This depth of awareness enables us to trust in an unseen, but very real, process that is working. Author Ken Wilber calls it "spirit in action." This intimate perspective on life gives us the authority and the confidence to trust that no matter how rough the going, no matter the external controls or blocks, they are not our hope or inspiration. Then, armed with this awareness, we can boldly assert ourselves through silence, quietness, participation, or bold declarations. The choice is ours.

The more we submit to this awareness and ownership of ourselves, the more our choices become characterized by wisdom, which is sound decision-making. Ironically, the more disciplined we become, the freer we are to live our lives according to our mission and purpose. As time goes by, we become more comfortable and sure-footed with our sense of self. With this internal congruity, we begin to see the same kinds of alignment in our outer world. This is when we become aware that we have exchanged anxiety and dependency (addictions) for awareness, alignment, and authenticity. At this point we become sexual partners who are ready to also be lovers in the truest sense of the word.

Questions for Reflection

1. To what degree do you take time to become aware of your own self-talk?
2. What words would you use to characterize your self-talk today?
3. Has the nature of your self-talk remained similar or the same throughout your life, or has at changed at certain points? If the latter is true, what factors might have contributed to these changes in your self-talk?
4. List specific benefits that you can see happening if you were to become more aware and intentional with your self-talk.

Affirmation

The first way I bring love into my life is through self-love, which I cultivate first and foremost through the self-talk or messages I send to myself each day. I have the power to change my self-talk and to send new and affirming messages to myself that proclaim the sacred and inviolable value of my being, a being that is filled with a presence, a beauty, and a goodness that cannot be granted or taken away by anyone. I am enough just as I am!

Day Twenty-Three

Develop Your Sexual IQ

Below is a short quiz. Some items are true; others, false. Please mark T (for true) or F (for false) by each item, and then read on to see how you score.

1. Sexuality is a natural physical act.
2. Healthy sexuality means zero anxiety, tension, fear, or apprehension.
3. Sexuality is an uncontrollable part of self.
4. Healthy sexuality requires that your sexual partner accept and affirm you as you are.
5. Basically sexuality begins at puberty.
6. Rich, robust intimacy requires a healthy sense of identity.
7. A very active sex life may accompany a low level of experienced intimacy.
8. Sexuality is among life's most profound routes to spiritual development.
9. Far more people have sexual experiences than have sexual intimacy.
10. Sexuality is as basic to life as is creativity and play.

Perhaps you noticed a pattern to the list of questions. But whether or not this is so, consider each of the items for the truth and/or myth that it describes. Taken as a whole, the first five statements suggest that sexuality is largely a matter of performance and goal attainment.

We expect that if we are more sexual, we will be more loved or even more lovely. In addition, we tell ourselves that if we are anxious about having sex, something must be wrong with us. The performance model is based upon a belief that sexuality is a set of skills that can be learned and mastered. It fails to acknowledge that our sexuality is an integral and complex part of being human that cannot be parceled out to discrete parts of our body, psyche, or behavior.

The second five statements are consistent with beliefs that our sexuality is created within us for our development, including our pleasure, cocreation, and attainment of fuller meaning and joy in life. From this second perspective, our sexual experiences take on the character of being potential teachers and guides toward fuller, richer lives, not being a burden of sins to bear, confess, and repent of.

Perhaps as you read and reflect upon the ten statements, you see yourself somewhere in the mix of some agreement and disagreement with both sublists. This is not unusual because it seems impossible or highly unlikely that any of us begin life as mature beings. Rather, we are a unique mix of on and off the mark. But how we approach our lives becomes predictive of how we develop.

By this latter comment, we mean that our beliefs about the meaning of our experiences will greatly influence how we continue to develop. If we believe that our sexuality is inherently good and that it affords us pleasure, then guess what, that tends to be consistent with our experiences. If we believe that our sexual experiences reflect our level of skill and/or goodness, then guess what? We begin to see our faults and to feel guilty if we perceive that we miss the mark. Thus we are some degree of bad.

Consider that, at its core, sexuality is life energy. As such, sexuality can fuel the fires of passion that, when filtered with wise and caring choices, lead to enriching, even ecstatic experiences. But this innate energy, when activated by appetitive desires and selfish aggression, too often leads to guilt, pain, isolation, and regret.

We humans, as free agents, choose our sexual paths. We create consequences, patterns, relationships, and ultimately life stories. We do this chapter by chapter. Unfortunately, if we do not awaken our consciousness soon enough, we lose large segments of our lives.

The good news is that it is never too late to learn. But to shift our life course requires several intentional moves to redirect our life patterns. We become resilient by the following practices:

1. Taking ownership for the quality of our lives.
2. Practicing a tenacity toward the truth of the "isness" in our relationships.
3. Setting our intentions for what we want to create in our relationships.
4. Disciplining ourselves to follow through on our commitments and hold ourselves accountable.
5. Maintaining a small accountability group with whom we are transparent and consistent.
6. Enrolling ourselves in some form of consistent, continuous learning projects or initiatives.
7. Owning it and expressing remorse if/when we realize we've been more self-serving than generous and/or giving in our approach to our relationships.

Add your own ideas to the list.

As you reflect upon today's lesson, consider how you can continue to develop your own sexual IQ. Your future is yours to design.

Questions for Reflection

1. To what degree do you feel you have taken responsibility for the quality of your life and your relationships, sexual and otherwise?
2. How intentional are you in your day-to-day relationships?
3. To what degree have you been honest with yourself or someone else about your sexual choices and the impact they have had on your own life and others' lives?

Affirmation

By continuing to develop my own sexual IQ, my sexual experiences and relationships will be richer, more intentional, and more capable of teaching me valuable lessons about myself and others.

Day Twenty-Four

Challenge the Status Quo

Before we discuss what it means to challenge the status quo, take a look at the statements below. Consider each one carefully. Then ask yourself, "Does this statement capture any of the messages I have heard or received from my culture?"

- Sexuality is shameful.
- Sex outside of marriage is the end of the marriage.
- When Mom is happy, everybody's happy.
- If a man doesn't get sex at home, he'll get it somewhere.
- It's a man's job to make his woman happy.
- Frequent sex is sign of a good relationship.
- Good sex will always end with an orgasm.
- A child raised in a religious community will abstain from sexual intercourse until after marriage.
- An unplanned pregnancy outside of marriage will ruin a woman's life.
- Women, because they are hormonal, can't be trusted as leaders.
- Marriage will give us all the love and sex we desire. It is a dream come true.
- Overweight women are not attractive to men.
- A single woman who has had multiple sexual partners is a loose or immoral woman.
- A single man who has had multiple sexual partners is experienced and macho.

- A woman who has been raped needs to understand that her choice of clothing may have contributed to her rape.
- Men cannot manage their sexual desires as well as a woman can.
- Workplace sexual relationships, when considered to be against company policy, will result more often in the woman being transferred or fired.
- The power hierarchy is based on masculine traits. Feminine traits don't hold as much power.
- Men don't have as many sexual insecurities about their bodies as women do.

Jaime, barely out of college, bright-eyed, hopeful, and very naive, thought she knew so much about life, love, and relationships. And sex, well, that was important, but it was all genital-focused. After all, her parents had married at eighteen and twenty-one years old, had children, and were still happily married. Jaime was certain they knew the secret to what it took to have a good marriage. During Jaime's adolescence, her mother would say, "If a man doesn't get sex at home, he will get it somewhere else." Thinking her mother was speaking for both herself and her husband, Jaime saw them as trying to prepare her for marriage. On the morning of Jaime's wedding, she was told this again by the female elders in her family. So, wanting a good marriage, she initiated sex constantly with her new young husband. Jaime worked hard to make a good marriage and to keep her husband home and happy. But within their first year of marriage, he stated that he wanted a divorce. He added that six months into his marriage he had started having sex with someone else. Additionally, he confessed that he had been pursuing other women ever since his marriage. Well, the advice or "truth" Jaime had been told was blown to smithereens. She had been operating on a false and completely incorrect assumption. She had not challenged the status quo offered by the women in her family. But, boy, it got challenged for her!

That was the first of many wake-up calls for Jaime. If the so-called truth she had been told could be so wrong, what other assumptions might be wrong? Of course, little things such as "Eat the crust on your sandwich because that's where the vitamins are" and "Don't masturbate or you will go blind" humorously popped up along with countless other assumptions that were also not true.

Challenging the status quo is not about destroying our culture or family systems. It's about asking for the Truth with a capital *T.* Growing up, we take it for granted that what our parents and society teach us is correct. Sometimes it is, but sometimes it is not. It is up to us to ask.

1. What is it that I am assuming about myself, this person, or this situation?
2. Is it really True?
3. How do I know it's True? Who told me it was true and made me believe it?
4. Can I be the one to decide what is True?
5. How can I know whether something is or is not True?
6. Where is my authority? Outside me in another person or organization? Inside me? Who decides how I am to make my sexual decisions and what those decisions will be? My family, church, synagogue, Bible study, reference group, political party?

Locus of control is a phrase we use to describe the location of our control, that is, our true center. If we all come from the same source, then each of us has access to the same source. But do we consciously access this source? Ask yourself: Do I frame my authority as external to me, or do I learn that something may be the right thing for you but not be what I need to do? I need to make my own decision from within, knowing what I am to do and when, where, how, and why I am to act.

Your answers may differ from mine. I can decide what is right and true for me. I can decide if the principles on which I have been making decisions are sound or not. When challenging the status quo, we must use discernment. Discernment, the ability to decide between truth and error, is a deeply internal learning process. Without it we are just challenging or being rebellious like a toddler or teen who digs her heels in and says no for the sake of saying no. We show that we haven't really found our voice yet. We can challenge the external authority or status quo. You and I can grow to recognize our own internal authority or inner alignment/balance.

Questions for Reflection

1. To what degree have you accepted, questioned, or outright defied the beliefs around sexuality promoted by society's status quo?
2. What status quo myths about sexuality have you ever held as true, and what effects on your own life or others' lives can you see from your belief in these ideas?
3. To what degree do you feel willing to question the status quo? What potential risks and/or benefits might you experience by questioning some of the sexual myths held by many in our society?

Affirmation

I am committed to becoming more aware of the myths and stereotypes around sexuality that are promoted by my society's status quo. Moreover, I am committed to speaking up and taking action against the perpetuation of these myths and becoming someone who makes decisions based not on an external authority but on my own growing internal wisdom.

Carefully Choose Your Close Circle

Carefully choose your close circle, your daily, most intimate community.

Just as emotions are contagious, so are attitudes and outlooks on the world. Much like a virus spreads, our outlooks and habits spread out to affect others, changing us and them at the same time.

This is why if you spend time with crooks, you become a crook and why if you spend time with saints, you become more loving. It is because our learned behaviors and attitudes can act like viruses, spreading widely, infecting others with our worldview or perspective.

Our sexual values are the same, mutating and spreading exponentially throughout our culture and beyond, changing how people see and live their sexual energies.

Right now, right where you are, put your sexual values, beliefs, and behavioral patterns under a figurative microscope. What do you see? What you see will spread as you express your sexuality.

What sexuality virus are you strengthening and spreading? How can or will you infect others?

Viruses are very difficult to control or stop, so think carefully: what virus do you want to contract and spread?

Picture yourself going viral sexually. Each person with whom you are sexual or with whom you communicate a sexual message becomes a node that carries the virus outward. Your virus is powerful. You are paying forward your sexual message with each sexual encounter.

You decide: is the sexual code that you spread one of love or fear?

Questions for Reflection

1. How carefully have you chosen the circle of people to whom you are closest in your life?
2. What words would you use to characterize this circle of people? Do the words you choose stay the same for everyone, or would you describe each relationship differently?
3. Consider and reflect on two or three examples of viral messages pertaining to sexuality that you have received or sent to the people in your inner circle. Were these messages sent through words, acts, or attitudes, and what were their effects on your life?

Affirmation

I am responsible for choosing my own inner circle, and I am aware of the vast power each of us has to influence others through our choice of attitude/thoughts, words, and actions. Therefore, I choose to associate with people who have a positive and healthy attitude toward their sexuality and toward the role that sexuality plays in all our lives. Moreover, I commit to being a person who sends positive and healthy messages about sexuality to the people I love and care about most.

Replace Your Sexual Fears with Your Legitimate Sexual Story

Call out your sexual fears so that you can replace them with your legitimate sexual story.

David, a successful businessman in his midfifties, finds himself recently divorced. Friends are trying to set him up with single women. Consistently, David finds excuses not to be available. He knows he's afraid, but he's reluctant to risk his worst nightmare of not being able to perform.

Across town lives Sandy, an attractive seventy-year-old widow. Sandy and her husband had an active sex life. In fact, her husband, Rodney, had a massive heart attack while they were having sexual intercourse. Rodney died on the way to the hospital. Sandy feels guilty and tells her best friend that she is interested in dating but is afraid that whomever she dates will want to have sex—and she doesn't know how to navigate the whole dating experience.

Depending upon our sexual history, we will most likely have one of two postures toward life. We will have learned to trust, or we will mistrust our ability to navigate effectively in this world. And depending upon our choices, we may tend to become more fearful and anxious, leading us to become more defended and cautious, or we will become more resilient and hardy.

If the pattern of fear is the one that we adopt, our life story takes on tones and themes quite different from those taken on if we choose trust, encouragement, and anticipation of more good things to come.

Living with fear can be a terrifying thing, so we learn to keep fear at bay, not acknowledging that its origin is within. So while fear blocks our life energy and hinders the flow of our souls, we rarely call it out as the culprit that it is. This occurs in the sexual arena just as it does in any other arena.

Think about some of the consequences of choosing fear over participation:

- Because of fear, you wait for your partner to initiate.
- Fearful, you construct defensive walls to protect yourself from perceived threats.
- Fearing oppression, you submit before it is demanded you do so.
- Fearing ridicule, you overcompensate with what you think are "good" and "safe" choices.
- Fearing rejection, you avoid new relationships.
- Fearing making a mistake, you defer to others and follow them.
- Fearing punishment, you become tediously compulsive about keeping the rules and laws.

Among the most damning consequences of this fear-based living are the lives defined by isolation, crippling addictions, and endless, joyless days that result in patterns of compulsive attempts to change things and that alternate with episodes of despair.

Not realizing that we are our own enemy, we continue to deceive ourselves and to look for someone outside ourselves to love us enough to make life worth living. This one self-deception tops our list of blocks to true joyful living. And just as this principle is true in other arenas of our lives, it is definitely so in our sexual life space.

Once we admit that we are fear based in our motivation, we can face our fear and begin on the route to healthy, love-based motivation. When we identify this dynamic between fear and life energy, we are free to begin making real lasting changes.

If we identify our sexuality, particularly our sexual practices within our relationships, as a top priority for healthy living, then we open a door that can take us to additional pathways toward wellness. This means that our sexuality, as it becomes more balanced, caring, and relationship affirming, becomes our path toward more dynamic living in multiple areas of our lives.

We turn fear into life-affirming actions by way of the following choices and actions:

1. We name our fears instead of deny them.
2. We realize the losses that we incur when we let fear drive our choices.
3. We replace these fears with visions of our true desires.
4. We set specific intentions with dates and particulars that define traits to be achieved.
5. We imagine our new choices, relationships, and levels of well-being.
6. We appreciate how the gift of our sexuality is taking us to new heights (or depths) of living!

As the older mentor Saint Paul taught his young protégé Timothy, "Perfect love casts out fear."

As we say, Trust your new, robust sexuality to take you to invigorating, playful, affirming new ways of being and of relating! Fear no lack of learning potential!

Questions for Reflection

1. To what degree and in what instances has fear guided your decisions pertaining to your sexual relationships?
2. To what degree does fear continue to guide your decisions related to your willingness to be vulnerable in relationships and to express your authentic sexuality?
3. Can you imagine a time or a moment when you experienced your sexuality in a full, robust way without fear? What words would you use to characterize yourself and your self-image and self-talk at this time? Can you imagine these characteristics as part of your essential self, not bound to acceptance or approval by any particular person?

Affirmation

I give myself permission to release my fears and to trust that I can live a rich and joyful life, one that includes vibrant sensory and sexual pleasure! My sexual well-being is mine to enjoy, to nurture, and to value. While I savor sharing my sexuality in thoughtful and generous ways with my partner, I begin with gifts of unconditional love and validation to myself. Every day I remember that the more I love myself, the more love—and pleasure—I must share!

Use Your Sexuality to Mature Your Love

Set your expectation to use your sexuality to mature your love, which is your birthright.

During the previous days, we have said that our sexuality is a birthright, a freedom, a joy, an energy, and more. And indeed we view sexuality as among our most precious birthrights. But on this day, we are reminded that our sexuality is best when it is lived in service to a higher purpose—that specific purpose being to mature our capacity to love!

Throughout the ages and across all cultures, wise teachers agree: love is paramount. Without love, we wither. We become cynical and destructive, often dying in heart and head before we die in body. Thus it behooves each of us to be students of both sexuality and love.

Today, ask yourself this: "How do I define love?"

And when you have this definition in mind, ask this second question: "Knowing me as he or she does, would my sexual partner describe me as loving?"

Several factors influence the extent to which we choose love over fear. Among these is our understanding of the nature of love. According to author Erich Fromm in *The Art of Loving*, love always entails four characteristics:

1. Care—actively wanting and acting to create growth and better living for someone important to us
2. Responsibility—maintaining a state of readiness to respond to another person's needs as they present
3. Respect—the capacity to see one as he or she is without judgment or manipulation, while at the same time wanting the person to realize his or her full potential
4. Knowledge—possessing a deep and comprehensive grasp of who a person is.

We often speak of three kinds of love: eros, phileo, and agape. Eros is love that springs from personal desire or passion; phileo is companion/friendship love; and agape is the deep empathic and compassionate service toward another that may involve sacrifice. Actually these three types of love speak more to the objects or audiences who will be loved more than to the nature of love itself.

As a sexual person, which of the following items describe you?

1. Faithful to commitments
2. Patient with my partner and myself
3. One who has a sustained, attentive focus on doing what is best for the other person
4. Disciplined in myself as way of committing to be my best self for my partner
5. Freely giving "grace" to the other, not as a condition of it being earned

The foregoing five characteristics are consistent with the required practices listed by Fromm when he discusses love as an art, meaning that love is both theoretical (meaningful) and applied (practiced).

As you infuse your sexuality with love, you set the stage for more love in all areas of your life.

Remember that we become that which we are in thought and action. In addition, if we treat those we love as we want to be treated, we draw more of that same type of energy to ourselves.

Lived this way, our sexuality truly becomes one of our most delightful languages of love.

Questions for Reflection

1. To what degree do you think your sexual experiences and choices are being connected to the energy of love?
2. In what ways can you imagine sexual love being enriched not just by erotic love but also by phileo and agape love? Picture specific enhancing changes in your relationships that you see happening as you mature your sexuality.

Affirmation

My sexuality affects my capacity to love. At the same time, I acknowledge that it is love within me, calling me forward to mature my sexuality. The two are intertwined! My sexuality is matured and enriched by the beautiful power of love. My sexual experiences will be richer, more blissful, and more grounding. Now I perceive the beauty of life, my partner, and myself more fully!

Day Twenty-Eight

Develop Your Capacity to Be an Intimate Sexual Partner

We are not alone. Instead, we are connected. We are connected along the time continuum, past–present–future. We are connected in our thoughts, feelings, and behaviors. We are connected physically, too. Within thirty minutes of being in a room together, two people are exchanging air vapor with one another. And finally we are connected on the self–other continuum. There is no such thing as real separation. Have you ever seen a spiderweb at night? If you gently try to touch even one little piece of it, the entire web moves. That's how connected all of us are.

Throughout our lives, though, we have learned ways to create distance between ourselves and others, building walls between "us" and "them." Acting tough while holding our more tender selves inside, we become known, maybe even revered, for being rugged individualists. Sadly, too many individuals die lonely deaths, never having realized their capacity for intimacy. And yet people are longing to live in a space where they are not alone. People want to be known and to know because that is our spiritual DNA! *Intimacy* is where our hope lies. Intimacy is what bridges the distance between us and others.

When intimacy exists, two or more people share matters and/or space that is both very private and very meaningful to them all. There is an implicit agreement that each other's highest good will be honored and held with the utmost care, compassion, and competency that all involved are capable of.

On this day, we are speaking about sexual intimacy. All healthy sexual relationships are intimate, but not all intimate relationships are sexual. We define sexual intimacy this way: *sexual intimacy requires that a person contain his or her anxiety while expressing his or her authentic self. It is a learned capacity that requires vulnerability, curiosity, empathy, and humble audacity.*

Sexual intimacy is not for the faint of heart! Look at what it requires: vulnerability, curiosity, empathy, and humble audacity.

When we choose to make ourselves vulnerable to our sexual partner, we are willing to be undefended. And, yes, we are opening ourselves up to be wounded. When I allow you to know my tenderness, my desires, my insecurities, or my discomfort, you now have the power to judge me, humiliate me, or even reject me. There are no guarantees that I will be safe with you after my disclosures. But a strange thing often occurs. When people show us their weaknesses, the last thing we want to do is harm them. Our better side usually kicks in, and in response to their disclosures, we express care and compassion. And if we're honest, we will admit to resonating with their humanness. Their vulnerability does not bring out our defensiveness or killer instincts. At some level, we know what it's like to be in their skin (i.e., we have empathy). It's as if a junction or a synapse of union is created. Of course there are no guarantees of being accepted, and a betrayal after being vulnerable can be the most wounding thing of all. But without taking the risk of being known at a deep level, only a superficial relationship can be sustained. This is how sexual intimacy gets built.

We're here to learn and to grow into our full sexual capacity. This requires skills. Here are some key skills that are tools for the journey:

- self-awareness
- self-acceptance
- self-joy
- self-soothing ability
- self-discipline
- play (innocent)
- initiating play with our partner
- honesty
- respect
- gratitude
- willingness to contribute to sexual growth
- questioning
- tenacity toward the truth
- speaking the truth with kindness and respect
- bravery when it's risky
- transparency
- letting go of the need to control
- forgiveness
- expecting miracles
- using memories to benefit the present and future
- passionate desire to add value that transcends one's self
- laughter
- wise decision-making
- creation of coherent life patterns

In a nutshell, what is asked of us if we truly want depth-level intimacy is *humble audacity.* This is not the same thing as acting with gall or nerve, which could be defiant, retaliatory, resistant, impudent. Humble audacity is a posture of kindness and sensitivity, knowing that because we come from the same source, I am no better (or no worse) than you. I recognize that what I do to you, I do to myself, and thus I treat you as I would want to be treated. So I step out and take bold risks to up our sexual connectedness.

Questions for Reflection

1. To what degree do you feel you have experienced genuine intimacy with a sexual partner, meaning that you were able to contain or manage your own anxiety enough to express your authentic self?

2. List four or five of the skills listed earlier that contribute to your showing up more specifically to pleasure your sexual partner.

3. Recall experiences of genuine sexual intimacy: how did these experiences manifest your or your partner's capacity to feel and express empathy, curiosity, vulnerability, and humble audacity?

4. How do you imagine that your future experiences might be different or enhanced if you were to grow in your sexual intimacy skill set?

Affirmation

I recognize that as a precious human being, I am designed to desire and have real sexual intimacy! Sexual intimacy is a challenging, but infinitely rewarding, experience that I commit to cultivating in my day-to-day life by consciously choosing to develop my own self-management skills and to open more and more to my capacity to be curious, empathic, vulnerable, and more deeply true to myself and my partner.

Day Twenty-Nine

Use Wisdom in Sexual Decision-Making

Healthy sexuality is spontaneous. Much like the wind, it is completely mysterious and yet distinctly principled and ordered. Thus it takes *wisdom* and *integrity* to live our sexuality well instead of having it, at a minimum, distort our lives or, at the worst, destroy our lives.

What is *wise* sexuality? First, let's define wisdom. The essence of wisdom is sound decision-making.

The nature of wisdom is distinctly different from the nature of knowledge. Knowledge suggests comprehension of information along with shrewd and careful analysis, leading to the synthesis of information and analysis in order to make decisions that both prevent disappointing results and further the attainment of goals.

Wisdom embodies knowledge plus perspective. Values, intuition, and compassion for all persons who stand to be affected by the decisions are weighed as a decision is made. Wisdom often comes only through years of consistent practice. It embodies active learning through self-study, along with collective reflection and dialogue.

A hallmark of wisdom is the integration of spirit with ego, meaning that self-interest does not edge out the deeper spiritual/heart and soul concerns inherent in any decision.

Wise sexuality is sexuality that suggests each of the following points:

- a concern for all parties
- a readiness to accept all consequences
- a conscious awareness and presence while engaged in sexually oriented behaviors
- a respectful but also playful enjoyment of sexuality
- a continuity across both sexual and nonsexual encounters that maintains the integrity of the whole relationship
- an absence of either shame or guilt related to one's sexual decision-making
- an atmosphere of joy, love, and delight
- an element of sacredness or reverence that results in careful, skillful, and joyful expressions
- an energizing effect upon each party that lingers beyond any distinct encounter
- a kind and considerate respect for boundaries that maintains privacy and yet paradoxically allows for the other to introduce new modes of experience that may change the modes of experience and/or communication.

Questions for Reflection

1. Considering your sexual relationships, how well do you think they reflect the criteria of wise sexuality listed earlier?
2. What concrete steps can you begin to take to ensure that future decisions you make regarding your sexuality are grounded in genuine wisdom? List five or more ways that wisdom is guiding you toward greater sexual maturity.

Affirmation

Deep wisdom is available to me always, revealing itself when I invite it into my mind and heart with great appreciation and responsiveness. Today I seek only a mature and wise sexuality. When I move and act from wisdom, I, along with many others, am blessed beyond all measure.

Seek to Know Yourself as Full Embodiment of Spirit

Society still overidentifies sex with sin. In some ways, this is no wonder. Pornography has become a billions-of-dollars-a-year industry that seizes upon the exploitation of our bodies as if our bodies were separate from the sacred. But wasn't our physical form created by the Source, by the divine? Our personalities and bodies are very sacred, so very holy, yet they are vulnerable and intricate. The historic King David wrote, "We are fearfully and wonderfully made." We are to take care of our bodies and personalities, respect and even love both. To be human is to be divine. Spirit and form are already one; from the beginning they were joined together. We are not to separate them.

Pornography is a diminishment of that sacred union, of what is holy and of spirit. Pornography does not acknowledge spirit, our lasting value, and it excuses us from any sense of stewardship or responsibility, suggesting there are no lasting consequences. Pornography makes us less human, not more human.

Sexuality is our bridge, our connection, the dance between our spirit and our form. It is what awakens us to the truth that spirit and body are joined together from the beginning, at the very least from when we take our first breath. And what a magnificent dance our sexuality is! This is our libidinal life energy. It's creative, abundant, infinite, and life-affirming. We have the incredible job and the awesome responsibility of releasing this magnificent energy, our sexuality, out into the world.

Problems arise, though, when our sexuality is reduced to simple genital-focused activity. How-to sex manuals, flirtation, foreplay, positions preferences, toys, and games all have a place, but sex itself is not the end-all, be-all of our sexuality. So why would we want to reduce our sexuality to sexual acts? Sexuality is much more than that. Perhaps we reduce our sexuality to sex only because we have no deeper understanding of how *sex is only one expression of sexuality.* How we dress and use color and/or fashion; how we cook with focus while sipping a glass of wine then savoring each bit of our creation; how we can have deep belly laughs at ourselves and the irony of our life experiences; how we paint or create new works of art; how we are humbled with awe at the colors of fall or the mountain meadows amid the backdrop of snowcapped peaks; ways we come up with new inventions; how we sing in the shower or, better yet, while we are driving; how we dance when no one is around; how we write from our heart and intuition; how we do our jobs daily; and how we approach sex are all expressions of our sexuality. Each of these is one of the many expressions of spirit and body as one. The two vibrate in every cell of our being. The good news is that this is our birthright and continues in us and through us until we take our last breath.

For a visual of how spirit and flesh are joined and work together, consider the following diagram, "Model of a human being," by Dean Schlecht. Think of this diagram as an hourglass. There are four parts to this model of a human being:

- Spirit / Creator / God / Oneness / Source / Ground of All Being. Our essence and origin sits at the base of the hourglass. This is from where we come. The idea here is that we did not create ourselves; we come from something greater. This something greater permeates us.

- Psyche/soul—nonphysical essence. This is the part of us that exists before our bodies are formed. It holds our particularities, the nonphysical essence of who we really are at the core, our truest identity. Spirit flows through this part of us, carrying our uniqueness into our flesh.
- Form: body and personality (flesh). This is the physical part of us, our ego nature, the "me" one typically identifies with. But this form, this flesh, is what carries spirit out and into our world and interacts with our world.
- Environment. This is the world in which we live, interact, work, and travel. It also includes the relationships we have.

Model of a human being
Environment (our world)

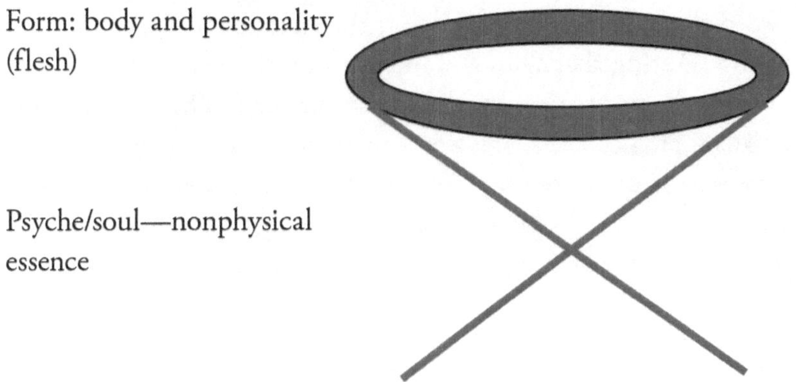

Spirit / Creator / God / Oneness / Source / Ground of All Being

Used with permission of Dean Schlecht.

When all is flowing smoothly, spirit is flowing through us, through our essence, and into our flesh/form/ego, thus enabling us to connect with our world. Our personality and body can choose to block this flow and to act devoid of spirit. Sadly, people will at times make that choice. Better, though, is that we acknowledge the spirit and body connection and bring the two into alignment, thereby owning the enormity of our sacredness.

What does this have to do with sexuality and relationships within the sexual realm? Theologian Martin Buber's book *I and Thou* talks about three kinds of relationships: I–it, I–you, and I–thou. The I–it relationship would seem to perceive and treat the other person as if he or she were an object whose existence was only for our pleasure. There's no sense of reciprocity within this relationship. The I–you relationship acknowledges the other person as more than an object and as having needs and wants. But the I–thou relationship recognizes and treats both oneself and the other person as the holy, sacred, spirit-filled, flesh beings they are.

The following model shows how our individual unique life span as two distinct periods. Period one is the time spent in our mother's womb. During that short 8-9 months our physical bodies develop to carry the spiritual essence placed at our cores. The second period begins at physical birth. It is a psychospiritual gestation during which time we mature into full awareness, acceptance, and actualizing of our life's best ways of being. The tragedy or loss is when we abort the process or never awaken to its full capacity and freedom.

Model of physical and psycho-spiritual gestation

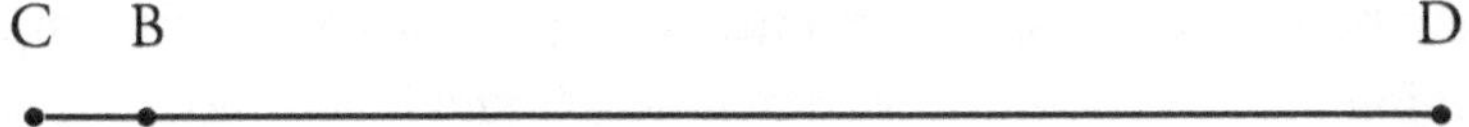

C—Physical conception, line between C and B is time in mother's womb

B—Physical birth, begins Period Two which is what we think of as our life span

From physical birth to physical death is psycho-spiritual gestation.

D—Physical death but also spiritual birth/transformation to "the other side"

We are not to separate the two, spirit and form. Through our radically mature sexuality, our body, personality, and spirit are one. Part of us already knows this. Consider: why do we scream "Oh God!" as an orgasm occurs?

Questions for Reflection

1. Consider the ways in which your body and your spirit are connected.
2. When has your spirit spoken to you through the sensations of your body? What words would you use to describe this experience?
3. Likewise, when have sensations in your body awakened an awareness of your spirit?

Affirmation

My body and my spirit are one. As I grow in sexual wisdom, this union of body and spirit becomes more harmonious, more beautiful, and more apparent to me and to others. My sexual decisions, while distinctly conscious and intentional, are also more relaxed and erotic.

Day Thirty-One

Commit to a Daily Practice that Will Strengthen and Renew the Sacred Bond between Your Body and Your Spirit

One of life's most invigorating symbols and rites of passage is marriage. The consummation or completion of this holy rite is the sexual union where those who were two become one.

Here is where we've come full circle. We began with the acknowledgment that our sexuality is as natural as breathing but not nearly as automatic. In fact, we've established that one of the most important tasks of our development is the conscious awakening and maturing of the intimate, mysterious, empowering relationship between our human and divine realities.

As we prepare to enter this space, we take comfort in remembering how world-class leaders in growth and development have presented scientific and theoretical evidence of the power of prayer and meditation. Internationally recognized physician Dr. Larry Dossey has published a book asserting the healing benefits of prayer. The Dalai Lama and teachers like Pema Chodron speak to large international crowds on the virtues of meditation. Similarly, the benefits of meditation have been demonstrated in scientific studies so many times that medical schools now require that physicians in training learn meditation skills as a valid form of treatment for medical illnesses.

Meditation enables us to access the place beyond the daily stresses, chaos, thoughts, and anxieties, often called the "monkey mind." Can't you just picture monkeys jumping branch to branch, tree to tree? Through meditation, we willingly stop and still our minds so that an opening to the divine is created. If you are not familiar with meditation, there are many good books and teachers on this subject. Check both onsite and online sources.

Prayer, while similar to meditation, is more initiatory. We speak with words or with our hearts of that which we are experiencing or desiring. Prayer is communication with God, the Source, the divine—however you wish to name or frame this presence. It can be a pouring out of our hearts, our worries, our gratitude.

You may be aware that prayer and/or meditation can take many forms. There is body prayer, a practice during which one creates movements to express one's interpretation and/or experience of what one is reading, thinking, and/or feeling. There is centering prayer in which one sits quietly and allows the spirit within to voice what is emerging from one's depth.

In terms of meditation, there are multiple forms, from silent breathing, harmony with a natural rhythm, to intentionally using daily routine types of tasks as if they have deeper meaning. For example, doing one's dishes can be a time for expressing gratitude for one's food and one's capacity to share a meal and for being able to create a clean and organized space in preparation for an upcoming meal.

We encourage you to explore how prayer and meditation can become an enriching part of your world. What is essential is your commitment to rediscovering, renewing, and strengthening your awareness of the connections within yourself and with your sexual partner in an unending presence and union with your Creator. Without a daily practice of slowing down and listening to wisdom, it is all too easy to lose sight of this connection and to fall prey to old temptations of living life through compulsions instead of through presence and purpose.

Questions for Reflection

1. How much have prayer and/or meditation been a part of your daily life up until now?
2. If prayer and/or meditation have been a part of your life, what impact do you think they've had on the quality of your life, especially your relationships?
3. In what ways might cultivating a daily practice of prayer and/or meditation impact your appreciation for living life as a sacred spirit inhabiting a beautiful human body?

Affirmation

I acknowledge and give thanks for the union between my spirit and my body. Desiring to experience this union more fully, I commit to a daily practice of prayer and/or meditation as an essential means by which I can remember, renew, and reharmonize these precious aspects of my being.

Beyond the Thirty-One Days

A Sample Prayer

The following prayer addresses the development of a fully conscious, loving relationship.

> I would like to think you have also prepared my lover, but I do not know. And I do not control. This I know: I come shedding all pretense or demands.
>
> I come to dance freely, passionately, unadorned and unarmed with fake jewels, but dressed in luxurious natural oils, sparkling with anticipation, alert with desire.
>
> Before we were enemies, competing for more, dancing in coy sparring battles to determine who was superior and who inferior—one up, one down, oh no, face-to-face, but still holding back. Safety with satisfaction. The expense, well, surely not for me. Oh no, I keep myself unencumbered, ready to leave at the moment I sense any hesitation on your part. But now, ah, sweet now,
>
> Now is different. I am peace. I am joy. I am strength. I am initiating this dance, never, my love, to hurt you. But this you must know:

What I bring is precious, the oils with which I desire to bathe your very soul and your precious vessel. Before I pour them upon you with erotic fervor, this is the one thing that I require, even fiercely require, of you:

You must meet me naked, unashamed, still, eyes wide open, mouth agape with dripping desire. You must want me. You must move your hands to absorb my body. You must assert yourself as a brave warrior, leaning into the wind. You must pause, stilled in awe of this wondrous circle in which we are one with light, fire, and piercing, erupting creativity.

Only then are we in sync. Only then are we ready to approach the altar. Only then do we, in sacred unison, declare, "Oh God!" "Where two are gathered, there I am," says God, in your midst. Oh my God! For this I have waited my whole lifetime. May I never again settle for less!

Amen, and amen, and amen!

We hope that you have enjoyed this month and that you are now ready to reread the field manual and let the work truly begin as you commit, setting your intentions and scheduling your days to live for the rest of this life span as a brave and bold, yet soft and caring, warrior for sexual healthiness in service of holistic wellness.

As you begin this next chapter, the one that you shall write, know that we wish you much learning, joy, and divine presence.

References

Burton, Sir Richard, trans. *The Kama Sutra of Vatsyayana*. Barnes & Noble, 1995.

Carter, Jimmy. *A Call to Action: Women, Religion, Violence, and Power*. New York: Simon & Schuster, 2014.

Chang, Jolan. *The Tao of Love and Sex*. New York: E. P. Dutton, 1977.

Crooks, Robert and Karla Baur. *Our Sexuality*, 8th ed. Boston: Wadsworth Thomson Learning, 2002.

Dick, Kirby (filmmaker). *The Invisible War*. Chain Camera Pictures, 2012.

Eisler, Riane. *Sacred Pleasure*. New York: HarperCollins, 1995.

Eyler, David and Andrea Baridon. *More than Friends, Less than Lovers: Managing Sexual Attraction in Working Relationships*. Los Angeles: Jeremy P. Tarcher, 1991.

Feuerstein, Georg. *Sacred Sexuality*. Los Angeles: Jeremy P. Tarcher, 1992.

Flora, Carlin. "Just Friends." *Scientific American Mind* (January–February 2014): 30.

Fromm, Erich. *The Art of Loving*. New York: Harper & Row, 1956.

Helminski, Kabir. E. *Living Presence*. New York: Jeremy P. Tarcher / Putnam, 1992.

Katehakis, Alexandra. *Erotic Intelligence*. Deerfield Beach, FL: Health Communications, 2010.

Krebs, Christopher P., Christine H. Lindquist, Tara D. Warner, Bonnie S. Fisher, and Sandra L. Martin. "The Campus Sexual Assault (CSA) Study," conducted January 2005–December 2007 for the National Institute of Justice.

Martin, Colby. *Unclobber: Rethinking Our Misuse of the Bible on Homosexuality*. Louisville, KY: Westminster John Knox Press, 2016.

Massachusetts Institute of Technology. "Survey Results: Community Attitudes on Sexual Assault." October 27, 2014.

McCarthy, Barry. *Sex Made Simple*. Eau Claire, WI: PESI, 2015.

Newsweek. *Fifty Shades Phenomenon: Exploring a Sexual Revolution*. New York: Topix Media Lab, 2015.

Osho. *Meditation*. New York: St. Martin's Griffin, 1996.

Peck, M. Scott. *The Different Drum*. New York: Simon and Schuster, 1987.

Schlecht, Dean. Personal communication to L. Carlson. June 19, 2009.

Schnarch, David. *Passionate Marriage*. New York: W. W. Norton & Company, 1997.

Spong, John. *Living in Sin*. New York: HarperCollins, 1988.

Stover, Dawn (Ed). (2016) The Sexual Brain (Special Issue). *Scientific American Mind.* 25 (1) New York.

US Equal Opportunity Employment Commission. About EEOC: Outreach and Education. Washington (DC). Accessed October 24, 2019. www.eeoc.gov.

Wilber, Ken. *Integral Psychology.* Boston: Shambhala, 2000.